ATYPICAL PREMED

by Dr. Danielle Ward

Atypical Premed

By: Dr. Danielle Ward

First paperback edition January 2020

Book cover design by Sam Arts

Book interior designs by Illumination Press

Book interior formatting by Richard Sheffield

ISBN 978-1-7344555-0-2 (paperback)
ISBN 978-1-7344555-1-9 (ebook)

Printed in the United States of America
www.aspiringminoritydoctor.com

To My Loving Daughter, Tiana
May you never stop reaching for your dreams

TABLE OF CONTENTS

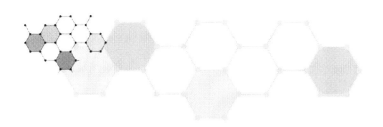

INTRODUCTION

Non-Traditional Students: You Are Not Alone

The decision to apply to medical school is not one that can be made easily overnight. It takes years of preparation to construct a decent application, and even then, acceptance is not guaranteed. The process is especially grueling for non-traditional students who do not fit the cookie-cutter mold of the thousands of students applying to medical school each year. As a three-time medical school applicant and former non-traditional student, I know all too well the difficulties and obstacles that come along with the decision to start on the path to becoming a physician.

I wrote this book with the intent to both guide and encourage students from all backgrounds who are interested in pursuing a medical career. Whether you are a single parent, changing careers, involved in the military, an older (or even younger) student, or involved in anything else that does not fit the typical view of an entering medical student—if you plan on applying to medical school, this book will have something for you.

My hope is that this book will serve as an excellent resource for those who do not know where to begin in their journey. It will be filled with advice, tips, and my own personal experiences in an attempt to show that anything is possible despite any obstacles that may be faced. I hope this book will inspire you and bring you that much closer to your dream of becoming a physician.

THE
NON-TRADITIONAL
STUDENT

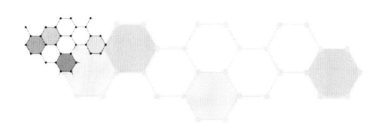

WHAT IS A NON-TRADITIONAL STUDENT?

Typically, a non-traditional medical student is one who did not enter medical school directly from college, but there are plenty of exceptions to the rule. I have met non-traditional students who entered college at a younger or older age than most students, and went straight to medical school afterwards. There are also students who consider themselves non-traditional due to life circumstances. There is no one complete and specific mold that defines a non- traditional student, but generally if you are older (or younger) than the average age of students entering medical school, have a family to take care of, or feel that you have a unique circumstance that makes you different from the average premedical or medical student, then you can consider yourself to be non-traditional.

Is being a non-traditional student a bad thing?

Absolutely not! As a non-traditional student, you will most likely bring something to the table that many traditional medical students might lack, and that is life experience. You might be leaving behind a career, but you will bring with you a multitude of skills learned and the ability to work and get along with many different types of individuals and personalities. You might be raising a family, but the ability to manage not only yourself, but the lives of the family members around you, shows that you already have a good foundation of time management, compassion, and leadership. You might even be an individual who, for whatever reason, had to take an additional year or two off after graduating from college. You could have applied to medical school and been rejected the first time around, confused about how the process worked and ended up applying too late, or you were on the fence about applying for other reasons. The point is, there are many things that can cause an individual to fall into the non-traditional student category, but it is not something that one should be ashamed of.

If you are a non-traditional student, embrace it!

Sure, you will have to face additional challenges that most traditional medical school applicants will not, and it can be disheartening to not have many people to relate to on your journey, but it will just serve to make you that much stronger.

Making the decision to apply to medical school is not easy for anyone, but if it is really what you want, then go for it. Do not get sucked into other people's ideas of what you should be doing with your life. If medicine is truly your passion, and you cannot see yourself doing anything else in life, then pursue it with full force. Not only will you be happier, but the end results will be that much more worth it.

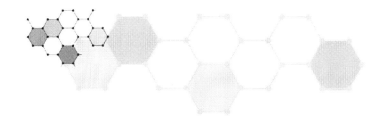

MY STORY AS A NON-TRADITIONAL STUDENT

There were many aspects that I believe made me a non-traditional student. The largest factor that identified me as non-traditional was the fact that I applied as a single mother who had been working ever since I graduated from college. I also considered myself to be non-traditional because I did not have the typical statistics (GPA, MCAT scores, etc.) of accepted applicants.

I graduated from a state university in December 2009 and started working full-time in research a few months after that. Fast forward to almost four years later, and I was still working full-time at the same institution. My research was somewhat medically-related, and allowed me to stay up to date with medical advancements, so I wasn't completely out of the loop when it came time to start medical school.

I first applied to medical school in 2008 and was rejected. After graduating and having one year of research under my belt, I applied again and got the same result. I knew that my GPA was a huge factor in my rejections, and the student loan companies were killing me with repayment fees, so I decided to enter into graduate school. This was not easy due to the fact that I had a GPA below a 3.0 and I also needed to work full-time to support my child. I researched possible online programs, and I was able to find an actual brick and mortar institution that offered graduate degrees that could be taken completely online. Although I did not meet their minimum requirements for matriculation, they allowed me to take two courses under a probationary status. When I aced the courses, I was then able to officially matriculate into the program. The program was extremely hard, but so worth it and I am glad to have made it through. I entered into medical school with a master's degree under my belt, and an excellent GPA to go along with it. This gave me an extra boost of confidence that I had what it took to succeed.

Being a single parent made me non-traditional because unlike other students, I did not only have myself to worry about in medical school. As an undergrad, I worked two jobs and attended school full-time in addition to being a single parent, and I believe it really impacted my grades in a negative fashion. Because of this, it was extremely important that I set up a support system prior to entering medical school so I could avoid some of the same obstacles.

The funny thing is that even though I was a non-traditional student, I think it actually helped me a lot in the long-run. I know what it is like to have to juggle finances, school, a child, and everything else that comes in between. I also had a few years to really take the time to enjoy life and have fun from time to time, so I didn't feel like I was missing out during my years as a medical student. I knew without a doubt that medicine was something I wanted to pursue, because I pursued other things, and something about it always called me back. In a way, I consider my four gap years as being a mini-vacation. I have awesome memories to look back on, and I was ready to pursue the next chapter of my life. They say your 20's are your best years, so I guess I'm kind of glad that I had the chance to experience many of the things that my traditional counterparts had not. Plus, I got to enter into medical school with a little more age and wisdom.

With that being said, my biggest advice for non-traditional students is to use the title as a strength and make note of the positives it has brought you. The rest of this book will focus on getting into medical school, and thus can be used by both non-traditional and traditional premedical students alike, but I hope these opening pages have reassured those who feel like outsiders in the process that you are not alone.

BECOMING A MORE COMPETITIVE APPLICANT

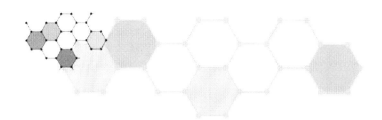

WHAT MEDICAL SCHOOLS LOOK FOR IN AN APPLICANT

There isn't one specific characteristic of a premedical student that guarantees acceptance into medical school. Most medical schools desire a well-rounded applicant who can stand up to the rigorous material and expectations that will occur over four years of training. They want a student who will be able to manage their studies while maintaining a good balance that allows for enjoyment outside of medicine.

Being a non-traditional student gives the advantage of being well-rounded as most of these individuals have already figured out a way to have a life outside of medicine. This is extremely important because medical training can be intense and all-encompassing. Not being able to have a balance outside of medicine can lead to depression, decreased performance, and other issues that medical schools try to avoid.

This section will address areas in which premedical students can become more competitive and well-rounded applicants. I will discuss topics such as desired grade point averages (GPAs), the dreaded MCAT, and extracurricular activities that medical schools look for in selecting applicants.

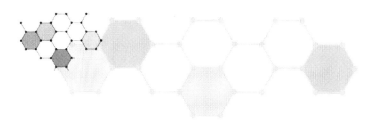

POST-BACC, SMP, OR ANOTHER DEGREE: WHAT'S RIGHT FOR ME?

If you are a non-traditional student who has been out of school for a while, or you are looking to bring up a low undergraduate GPA, you'll need to explore all your options for becoming the most competitive applicant possible. There are many options available to prove to schools that you will be able to handle the heavy course load that comes with medical school. The following will be a discussion of some of these options, so that you can best decide what will work best for your situation.

Post-Baccalaureate Coursework

A popular choice among many non-traditional students is to take undergraduate courses as a non-degree seeking student. This is commonly referred to as a post-baccalaureate program (post-bacc). Most medical schools will count these courses as part of the overall undergraduate GPA, so this could be a good way to boost your GPA. This method is also particularly useful if you were a non-science major during college, because it can be used to take all the required science pre-requisites in addition to increasing your science GPA. The science GPA is weighed most heavily by medical schools, so if you do decide to go the route of taking post-bacc coursework, make sure that it mostly consists of science coursework. Also, if you are a non-traditional student who already has an undergraduate degree in the basic sciences, pursuing a post-bacc will only be beneficial if you take upper-level advanced science courses.

For some students, pursuing a post-bacc might not be as beneficial. If you already have an undergraduate degree with over 130 hours, taking more classes may do very little to increase your overall GPA.

Also, as a non-degree seeking student, you will not be eligible for any federal financial aid, so you will have to either pay out-of-pocket or take out private student loans. When the high interest-rates associated with private loans and course fees are taken into account, this can prove to be a very costly path.

Special Master's Programs

Another great option for proving that you can handle the heavy course load of medical school is a special master's program (SMP). These programs typically last between 1 to 2 years, and they generally cover advanced science coursework. A few SMPs are linked to medical schools, and as a student you will be taking the same classes as a first-year medical student. Some of these programs also take place at medical schools, and allow you to take the courses right alongside current medical students. This is an excellent way to prove that you can handle medical school, and if you are interested in attending the medical school of the program you attend, then it provides a way to network and get to know the professors. Furthermore, these programs are covered by federal financial aid.

The only downside with SMPs (and pretty much any program) is that if you do not perform well academically, it can greatly diminish your chances of gaining an acceptance into medical school. SMPs are also a popular choice among many premedical students looking to increase their GPAs, so acceptance into some of the programs could be very competitive. Also, while there are many SMPs throughout the United States, there may not be one in your area. This may mean that you will have to relocate to pursue the program. This may not be feasible for some students.

A Second Bachelor's Degree

Some students decide that getting a second degree is a better option for them. A second bachelor's degree is probably most beneficial to students who previously obtained a non-science degree and/or previously did not perform as well. In this case, a second bachelor's degree would not only give them a science GPA to work with, but it would also work to increase their non-science GPA as well.

Unfortunately, pursuing a second bachelor's degree can prove to be very costly out of all the options due to the fact that you will essentially be paying for another four years of school. If you are a non-traditional student who has been out of school for more than a decade, this might not seem like a bad choice, but this commitment does not come with a guaranteed acceptance into medical school and it will take longer to complete than all of the other options listed here. If you have been in the workforce for a while, and you are looking to get an advance in your career as a plan B option, another bachelor's degree just might not be useful as most companies require a master's degree or higher in order to climb up the corporate ladder.

A Master's Degree (or higher)

Obtaining a graduate degree is another viable choice for making yourself a competitive applicant, but unfortunately it is not a common path for premedical students. Obtaining a master's degree was the path I chose to take to boost my competitiveness as an applicant, and it is what I credit to my acceptance into medical school.

Typically, it only takes 1-2 years to complete these programs, and a thesis-based program is not required if your only goal is to go onto medical school.

Some non-traditional students are career-changers, so they may already have a graduate degree when they decide to apply to medical school. If the degree is recent, then it may help boost your chances of gaining an acceptance, but in some cases you may still have to have current coursework that will prove your current ability to medical schools. Also, if medical school is your main goal, you will have to seek out programs that do not require the added time of completing a thesis. For non-traditional students who have more advanced graduate degrees, such as a PhD, there are medical schools with pathway programs specifically for non-traditional students of this type, so I highly recommend looking into this if it applies to you.

DO UPPER LEVEL UNDERGRADUATE COURSES REALLY HELP IN MEDICAL SCHOOL?

Sounds like the workload is super intense! Does it really help to have taken undergraduate classes like microbiology, immunology, etc.? Or are you referring to your master's level classes? It seems like a lot of people say not to bother with taking more science classes in undergrad because the focus and volume in med school will be very different... but I'm wondering if it's true?

I was first asked this question a few years ago, and I've found that it is a question many premedical students seem to have. The workload in medical school will be intense regardless of whether or not you have had previous exposure. I took anatomy and microbiology solely on an undergraduate level, and the exposure did help, but very little. Understanding the terminology is a huge part of anatomy, and without any previous knowledge, it can make things a bit harder once you hit medical school, although you will probably make out just fine. I previously took anatomy back in 2006 and retained very little of the information I was taught. What did help was being familiar with terms such as prone, supine, origin, insertion, etc. This was not taught to us in lecture in medical school, but instead it was provided as a very large word document full of common terms. Since I remembered these terms, I was able to spend more time learning and retaining the material than trying to understand what every other word meant. The same applies for microbiology. I took it again during my second term of medical school, and can say with almost hundred percent certainty that I retained less than one percent of the material taught in undergrad, but being familiar with it helped.

When it comes to classes I took in my master's program, I can say that they are super helpful! During the first term of medical school, practically every course (with the exception of anatomy) was brand new to me, and I actually had to force myself to really learn the material. During my second term, practically every single subject we covered (minus pathology) was taught to me in my master's program. In my graduate program, I focused more on learning than memorizing, and it paid off really well during my time as a medical student. I even felt like I had more free time because I got to skip the basics. Having graduated, I can also say that medical school is not more difficult than graduate school in the level of the course work. In grad school, I had to literally write out mechanisms in biochemistry and I needed to learn, what felt like to me, every single, small detail about a subject. Biochemistry is way more enjoyable when you only have to know the major steps and components of glycolysis, versus having to know and be able to draw out the complete mechanisms like I did in grad school.

So, what is it that makes medical school so intense?

THE WORKLOAD!

Pretty much what might have taken me a month or two of graduate school to learn, we covered in about two weeks or less in medical school. This pretty much applied to every subject, so imagine an entire month of maybe nineteen credit hours in undergrad, double that, condense it into one week, and you have how fast we covered everything in medical school. It can be extremely overwhelming, and enough to make even the brightest students struggle. The focus is also different, but only in the sense that everything in medical school is more clinically-oriented. This was a positive aspect to me though, because I felt like I was actually learning about stuff that was relevant to my goals as a future physician.

So, if you're currently a premedical student considering taking advanced science courses, my recommendations follow this paragraph. If you are not able to take some of these courses, please do not stress about it. Even if it means you will have to put in a little more effort than your peers, chances are that you will make out just fine with or without taking these courses beforehand.

Recommended Courses to Take Before Medical School

	Anatomy		Biochemistry
	Embryology		Cell Biology
	Histology		Genetics
	Microbiology		Immunology

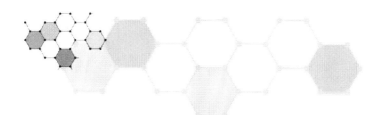

PURSUING AN ONLINE
DEGREE: MY STORY

As a non-traditional student and single mother, pursuing a post-bacc degree, SMP, or a second bachelor's degree were neither desirable nor financially feasible for me. Pursuing a post-bacc meant that I would have to pay out-of-pocket for classes I had already taken before getting my Bachelor of Science degree. As a biochemistry major with a minor in chemistry, there were very few advanced science courses that I had not taken (or re-taken for that matter), and it felt like it would be a complete waste of time. An SMP would have allowed me to take advanced classes, but with no guarantee of an acceptance to medical school and not much to show for it other than a certificate, I thought this was also a bad idea. I had a friend who completed an SMP at a medical school with hopes of being accepted, and despite earning good grades, unfortunately she was not. As a result, she did not know where she would go next. This further steered me from the SMP route.

I decided that it would be best to obtain a master's degree in biochemistry, but I needed something that was a bit more convenient. I worked full-time at a university doing research and as an employee I was entitled to six hours of classes each semester tuition-free (only three of those hours could interfere with work time). Unfortunately, most of the classes I needed to take were offered in the morning, and this was at the same time I was heavily doing experiments. I was also finished with my day by the time my daughter was dismissed from school, so evening classes were also out of the question.

I did an internet search for online graduate degrees, and it was extremely hard to find one in biochemistry. As a matter of fact, I think the school I attended may be the only one to offer an online graduate degree in biochemistry, or it was the first. Below, I will talk about pursuing a graduate degree online, and I will also address some of the questions I have been asked.

How were you able to enter into a graduate program without meeting the minimum GPA?

I entered into a Master of Science degree program at an institution where a 2.8 GPA was required, and for the Biology MS program at the same institution, a 3.0 was required. My undergraduate GPA was a few points below a 2.5 (yes, you read that correctly).

Thankfully, the school took pity on me and allowed me to enter into the program on probation. I had to take six hours of courses and do well. I accomplished this by starting during the summer semester with cell biology and biochemistry I. I passed each class with an A-, submitted my letters of recommendation, interviewed with the program director, and was finally accepted into the full Master of Science degree program.

How did you pay for the program?

For the first semester on probation, I was not considered to be a matriculated student for financial aid purposes. Because of this, I had to pay out of pocket for my first two classes. I took out a private loan for $5,000. This gave me enough money to pay for classes, books, and a new laptop. After I was accepted into the program, I qualified for federal loans, and that is how I paid for the remainder of the program.

I just want to note that if you can avoid taking out private loans, do not go that route. They are a horrible beast when it comes to interest rates and payment plans.

How do medical schools view online courses?

From what I have found, most medical schools do not accept online classes taken as an undergraduate student. My undergraduate degree was taken in the traditional way, so I did not need to worry about any medical schools rejecting my prerequisite courses. I did run into a few medical schools that do not accept any online coursework at all. Some of the people I spoke to in admissions held the belief that there is nothing better than actual classroom learning, but I think this is a completely backwards way of thinking. Everyone has a different way of learning, and I do not believe people should be penalized for doing what works best for them. (Interestingly enough, as a medical student, the majority of my lectures were recorded and streamed online, and I found learning at home still remained the best academic atmosphere for me.)

If you are concerned about whether or not a school will

accept your online coursework, the best thing to do would be to call them directly. Even though my transcript does not reflect that my courses were taken online, I fully disclosed this in my interview. For me, it would have been extremely hard to hide the fact that I lived and worked in the South but attended school in the North, so I put it all out there.

Are online classes easy?

ABSOLUTELY NOT! My online classes were the first time that I've ever had to work hard to get a good grade. With online coursework, you will constantly have to log in and engage in discussion, and there are assignments due every week. During one semester, I was literally submitting five to seven page essays every week, on top of discussion board posts, and essays in my other course. I also took a comprehensive exam in lieu of completing a thesis, and that was two days of pure torture. The funny thing is that in addition to my online classes, one semester I also took a regular class (virology) at the university where I worked, and it was so easy! I attended every class, zoned out, studied a day or two before each exam, and did great! The university course also gave multiple choice exams which is something you don't get very often in online courses, and I found these exams to be super easy. It really made me wonder where I went wrong in undergrad to have had such low grades.

To give an example of how hard online classes can be, I'll use my chemical thermodynamics course as an example. This was a calculus-based class that involved things such as deriving the Gibbs free energy equation and other well-known thermodynamics equations. It had been seven years since I had last taken calculus, so I had to use outlines to help me with integrations and everything else in the course. Also, because it was an online course, we had to figure out how to draw out all the equations using computer programs. It became so frustrating to me that I started handwriting everything and just scanning it in and submitting it. I am thankful that my professor allowed some of us to do this. The class also involved entropy and other calculations. There were definitely times I wanted to cry in the course, but I pushed through and made out with a B+. I learned a lot though, so I would say it was well worth it.

Online courses require a commitment like no other, and many people find that it is not the right route for them. I am more of a self-directed learner and do better when I have to take control of my learning. With traditional classes, it is easy to put everything off and just cram for exams, but online classes do not allow this. Also, I never really bought any textbooks during my undergraduate years because the questions mostly came from PowerPoint presentations. For my online classes, I bought and used every single required textbook. There were no lectures and only a few of my classes had PowerPoints, so I had to use YouTube and other sources to fully understand the material (which I still continued to utilize as a medical student).

Did you have to find a proctor for exams given online?

For the most part, exams consisted of essays and term papers. For classes that required mechanisms or equations, we would use computer programs to do this.

My pharmacology course had open-book exams that consisted of half multiple-choice, half essay questions, but even with the book right in front of me it was hard.

As a matter of fact, a lot of my courses had open-book exams, but I definitely had to know the material to answer the questions correctly.

The only time I did need a proctor was for my comprehensive exam. The exam consisted of six individual closed-book exams given over the course of two days. It was required for me to be able to officially graduate with my master's degree. For this, I was sent a really cool robot proctor. This thing took my fingerprint, had a 360-degree view of the room I was in, recorded sounds, and locked my computer from accessing anything other than the exams. It would be easier to cheat in a traditional classroom setting than with this thing!

Why I chose to get a full degree

I learned while applying to medical school that nothing is guaranteed. I wasn't going to spend thousands of dollars and not have much to show for it. I also figured that if I received a full master's degree, I could seek better employment opportunities due to having an advanced degree. I was prepared to take however long it took to try to get into medical school, but I had to be smart and think about my child as well. Also, research grants end and renewal is not guaranteed, so I wanted to make sure that when the time came I would be equipped with all the skills needed to move into another field, if necessary.

I no longer need to worry about that now, but it feels good

to have the extra credentials. The experience also helped me discover a lot about my learning habits, and was of great benefit to me during medical school.

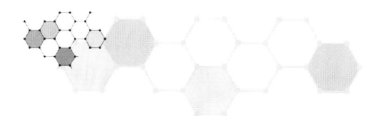

THE MCAT:
A PERSONAL REFLECTION

One of the questions I get asked a lot is what I did to prepare for the MCAT. Given that I took the exam multiple times, and the format has changed drastically since my time as a premedical student, I realize that I am probably not the best person to ask about this. Still, I figured it would be useful to write about my experience with this dreaded test. I have taken it four times, and have tried my best to remove it from my mind, but luckily I had a previously written blog post to help remember everything. I'll break it down into different sections to make it easier to read.

What resources did you use to prepare for the MCAT?

I first took the MCAT in 2008, and I only used Examkrackers at the time. I studied for it during the spring semester and I only took 14 hours of classes (one of my lightest semesters) which included microbiology, cell biology, physical biochemistry, a literature course, and physics lab. Looking back, it probably would have been better to wait until the semester was over and take an

August exam, but I thought May was when everyone took it. I did the 10-week at-home study program which you can find on their site, but with my course load and other obligations, I was not able to finish the program.

I ended up with a score of 21M (9VR, 6PS, 6BS), which is roughly equivalent to a 492 on the current MCAT scoring scale.

When I re-took the exam in 2011, I combined the Examkrackers material with The Berkeley Review (TBR). I will say that the TBR material was very in-depth and was great preparation. I also took the AAMC free practice test along with practice test 11 (and 2 others that I don't remember). I took the exam the first week of August and ended up with a 22Q (8VR 6PS 8BS). I was very disappointed with this score, but I'll get into why I think I scored this despite all my studying in a bit.

For my 2013 exams, I used Examkrackers, TBR, AAMC practice tests/assessments, and The Princeton Review Hyperlearning Science workbook (TPRH). For the first exam I took in July, I literally only used The Princeton Review Hyperlearning science workbook (my focus was on increasing my PS score). For the one I took in September, I would say that I relied mostly on the Examkrackers material, TPRH, and AAMC assessments. I do not think I practiced any verbal for either of the exams (I didn't practice in 2008, so I thought over-practicing was decreasing my score). For the July exam my score was 20 (6VR 7PS 7BS), and for the September exam my score was a 21 (7VR 6PS 8BS), which for current reference is around 491-493 on the current scale.

Thoughts on each resource

I think Examkrackers is pretty good if you have a firm understanding of the content. A major problem I had in undergrad was that I would just learn what I needed for the upcoming exams and then forget the material. I don't think I really developed a firm understanding of the material in undergrad to a point where I was able to connect and tie together all the different subject matter I learned.

I thought the Berkeley Review was pretty awesome, but you really do need to take the time to go through it. Unfortunately, this was time I did not have. I do remember taking the MCAT after using TBR, and I could have sworn that I saw some of the exact same material and passages. This is why I would recommend it. A suggestion for biology would be to only do the passages from TBR and use Examkrackers for content review.

The Princeton Review Hyperlearning science workbook was extremely helpful too. I was so focused on content review that I did not work out a lot of problems. Had I bought this book from the start, I probably would have scored a lot higher. I received it two weeks before my exam, and since my focus was only on physics, that is what I used it for. I increased my score by a point in that short timeframe, so I would definitely say that everyone should have this resource, although I am not sure that it is still in production or relevant to the new MCAT.

I think it goes without saying that the AAMC practice tests and assessments are extremely useful because they are made by the people who create the MCAT. Nothing beats true simulated testing conditions.

Why I think I did so poorly

Having too many other obligations and not focusing my energy on the test played a major part in some of my low scores. I also tended to over-study for the exams. For the MCAT that I took in 2011, I devoted 3 months to studying for the test and was doing at least 8-10 hours a day. I would come to work and study for most of the day in between doing research, and then I would come home and study until I couldn't take it anymore. It got to a point where I couldn't even think about the exam without becoming sick (literally). I also think that taking advanced science classes may have hurt me as well. The MCAT covers just the basics, and I think it is really easy to overthink things when you have learned more than what an introductory course teaches. I also could have benefitted from doing more practice problems instead of trying to re-learn the material.

Having taken all my medical board exams, I now know that I thrive and learn best from doing as many questions as possible. Back then, I was just too busy trying to learn the material that I never really learned the test.

Final Thoughts

Overall, I am so glad that I never have to worry about the MCAT ever again! I was prepared to do a January re-take when I got my scores back a week before I received an interview, but it was great having one less thing to worry about. Prior to attending medical school, I met other great physicians who admitted to scoring poorly on the MCAT and scoring high on the boards, and this was also true for some of my medical school classmates. This makes me wonder how indicative the MCAT is of one's success in medical school. I really wish the MCAT would not be regarded as highly as it is, but I guess that's life.

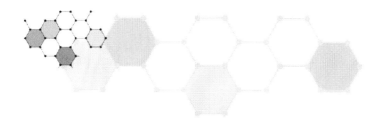

EXTRACURRICULAR ACTIVITIES (ECs)

With all the fuss that goes on about GPA and MCAT scores, a lot of people tend to forget another important aspect of the medical school application process: extracurricular activities (ECs). Some medical schools weigh these heavily because it shows that you can be a well-rounded student and balance multiple activities. It's easy to have a 4.0 GPA if the only thing you do is go to school and study, but it is way more noticeable if you can maintain a high GPA while being heavily involved.

In my case, I was extremely involved when I first started my undergraduate career, and I tried my best to maintain my activities even after I had my daughter. I will say that once I became a mother, it became a lot harder to keep up with my ECs, but I found a way to have meaningful employment that sometimes doubled as community service and work. A lot of students may have to work to support themselves or families, and I know medical schools take this into consideration as well. The point is to make sure you are always staying busy. You don't necessarily have to become an officer of an organization or do community service all the time, but if you can fit it in every once in a while, you should be good to go.

With that being said, below is a condensed list of the ECs I listed on my application (along with some commentary) so that you can get an idea of how they may have helped offset some of my low stats.

- **Research** – This is how I killed two birds with one stone. Research offered me paid employment, the chance to write abstracts and present posters out of state, and I got my name listed on a few publications. I had been doing research since junior year of undergrad. A lot of medical schools (and even residency programs once you're a medical student) want to see research experience, so if you're lucky enough to find a lab with money, this is a good route for a non-traditional student or someone who's been out of school for a while.

- **Hospital Volunteer** - I volunteered 4 hours every Sunday the entire year before I received an acceptance into medical school. I was in the Labor & Delivery department, so this mostly consisted of getting patients extra blankets, bottles, etc., and checking urine and diaper amounts. It was pretty low-key, so I used most of the time to study. Being in a hospital is also a good way to get the clinical experience that most schools want, and it lets you know if you really want to pursue medicine for the rest of your life. If you hate being in a hospital or if you don't like sick people, then you may decide another career path will work best for you.

- **Regular Volunteering** - Hurricane Katrina occurred during my very first semester of undergrad, so that is where my volunteering started. My school was one of the emergency centers for the state and since we were closed and classes cancelled, I spent a lot of long days and nights helping those being flown in. Clean-up volunteering was on-going for a few months after the storm.

  Volunteering can be anything that helps your community, so do not assume that it has to take place in a clinical setting.

- **Physician Shadowing** - I obtained over 200 hours of this prior to medical school just by spending every day one summer shadowing a DO. This took a bit of effort because I also had to work, but I somehow got it all in. In 2013, I shadowed another DO and got about 20 hours from this. Most osteopathic schools will require a letter from an osteopathic physician, and you are unlikely to get it unless you've spent some time with the person, usually in the form of shadowing.

- **Employment** - Outside of research, I held jobs that included teaching autistic children, working for the Battered Women's Program (BWP) legal office, being a coffee house barista, and even working for residential life on campus. The first two jobs doubled as community service in a sense, and my work for the BWP was one of my most meaningful experiences. As a single mother, I needed to make sure that my child was taken care of, but I really tried my best to have jobs that could benefit my medical school application as well. I wasn't afraid to serve coffee and work other odd jobs to make ends meet, so don't be afraid to do what you need to do to take care of yourself.

- **Organizations / Leadership** - During my undergraduate years, I served as an officer in a premedical organization, and I also was the Vice-President/Co-Founder of an on-campus HIV/AIDS organization. This took a lot of effort and it wasn't really feasible once I became a mother. I was involved until I couldn't be anymore though. Case in point: two weeks before I gave birth to my daughter, I was still actively involved in my organizational activities. I wore a sweatshirt to cover my huge belly, but I was out with a big smile on my face painting houses for the elderly.

- **Conferences / Presentations** - Whether I solely attended a conference or presented at one, I listed them all on my applications. Outside of those related to my research, I mostly attended conferences related to medicine, so in my opinion, listing them shows the schools that you really are interested. For presentations, I listed the conferences I attended and the ones I did not attend separately. Some of the research done in my previous lab was presented at international conferences, but I could not attend. If your name is listed on the abstract or poster, you can still list it and make a note that you were a contributor. Additionally, I listed the travel awards I received from some conferences.

That sums up my ECs. For one of my secondary applications I calculated the time spent on extracurricular activities and was surprised to find my volunteering and community service totaled more than 1500 hours.

For employment, I usually worked 25-30 hours per week. I know a few people who think they should list being a parent as an EC, but I am somewhat against this. While raising a child and attending school is a huge accomplishment, being a parent is a 24/7 job and not just an activity. I did mention the fact that I am a mother in my personal statement, but I left my activities section for everything else. I would suggest keeping track of everything you do from the time you start college, because there were quite a few things I forgot about and failed to mention in previous application cycles. This list can later be put into the form of a CV and used to give to your letter writers when the time comes.

RESEARCH AND PUBLICATIONS

Getting involved in research is not only a great way to enhance your medical school applications, but it provides invaluable skills that can last for a lifetime. I first became involved in research during my junior year of undergrad, and it was definitely not what I expected it to be at first. For some reason I thought I would just jump into experiments and come out with breakthrough research within my first month.

Never mind the fact that I had no previous research experience outside of a few class labs, and I still had a lot to learn.

My first few months of research involved stuffing pipet tips, washing equipment, and organizing specimens. Although I majored in biochemistry, I started off working in a genetics lab so I was exposed to a lot of new material that I had not yet learned. As time went on, I slowly began to learn about different genetics techniques, and I had the opportunity to apply some of the biochemistry methods that I had learned. I was soon doing Polymerase Chain Reactions (PCR), gene sequencing, electrophoresis, and an array of other things. It had its boring moments, but I always found everything extremely interesting. I was ecstatic when I was asked if I wanted to travel and present a poster at a summer conference, and this was also the time when I wrote my very first abstract. Attending conferences allowed me to become comfortable with speaking to people and presenting research. It also challenged me to learn more. There's nothing worse than being asked a question about your research and not having a clue what the answer is (and yes, I've had this happen to me).

I continued with the genetics research right up until the day before graduation, at which time I had to stop because the grant was only for undergraduate students :-(

Shortly after graduation, I applied for a position in a lab at the same university. It was a stretch since the position preferred someone with a graduate degree, but I applied anyway. The research involved parasitology and immunology, and I knew it would be a great way to spend a gap year or two before medical school. I was ecstatic when I got the job, and after four years, I only left because I was accepted into medical school and starting a new journey. Throughout my years in the lab, I was constantly amazed at how much everything continued to fascinate me, and up until the day I left, I was always getting to learn something new. I was able to work with blood, human parasites, and animals! I even got a chance to do my first chamber surgery around my third year in the lab, and for me there is no greater feeling than being able to cut open a living thing, suture it closed, and have it come back to life without any problems once the anesthesia wears off. I absolutely loved it!

To sum everything up, I wrote this chapter to say that if you are a premedical student and can get involved in research, then please do! It not only helps reinforce some concepts you will be taught in your classes, but it really does help develop critical thinking skills. Having a research background will cause you to question everything and look at material from many different standpoints. It also gets you out of your comfort zone and allows you to teach others about your work. It is one experience that I am glad that I have, and it can benefit you as both a medical student and future physician.

In terms of publications, although I had a few as a premedical student, this is not an absolute requirement for gaining an acceptance into medical school. It definitely adds a boost to your application, but do not be discouraged if you do not have the opportunity to have your name on a publication before entering medical school. For the more competitive specialties, publications are looked on favorably, and as a medical student, chances are you will have the chance to find many opportunities within your school. Lastly, a publication will always stay with you and be taken into consideration even if it was done as an undergraduate student or before starting medical school.

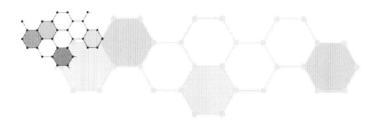

THE POWER OF NETWORKING

One thing I believe is most important in accomplishing any goal is networking and building relationships with those around you.

Everyone has something special to offer, and you never know what new things you can learn from the people around you. Don't be afraid to contact someone in the field that you are interested in and ask for advice. This is how I was blessed to receive many shadowing and volunteer opportunities in addition to the wonderful mentors that came along with them. It also helps to join various organizations.

One organization I highly recommend for all minority (and even non-minority) premedical and medical students is the Student National Medical Association (SNMA). I first became involved with this organization when I was a college freshman, and it opened so many doors for me. Every year the organization has an annual medical education conference, and this is where thousands of minority students gather to become empowered and educated in medicine. The first time I attended one of these conferences I was blown away at the thousands of minority medical professionals and students in one place. It was the first time in my life that I ever saw a large group of people who looked like me and had similar goals in life.

It was also the first time I was ever exposed to osteopathic medicine.

All of the conferences I attended were eye-opening experiences, and I had the opportunity to network with many people who I would have otherwise probably never met. Not only do these conferences have information for both premedical and medical students, but they have information on post-bacc and graduate programs as well. If you would like more information on the organization, feel free to check them out at www.snma.org.

I stayed involved with this organization throughout my medical school career, and it continues to benefit me even to this very day.

I even loved it so much that I served in various positions on both a chapter and national level and later went on to become the first osteopathic medical student to serve as National President of the SNMA. I was very involved as a medical student and joined multiple organizations, which served as great resources on my journey to becoming a physician.

On top of organizational involvement, carrying around a business card can help you with networking. It does not matter if you are a student. Just make sure that you have your contact information and your field of study. You never know when you might run into someone who can really help you get to the next level, and it is so easy to hand them a card rather than look for a pen and paper (or type it into your cellphone and forget it's there). In my opinion, having a business card is simply more professional.

Social media can serve as an excellent platform for

networking as well. Whether you have a Facebook, Twitter, LinkedIn, or other accounts, it is important to keep your information current and professional. I have oftentimes not been able to find an e-mail address for someone but have had access to their Facebook page. It never really hurts to contact someone that may be able to help you or offer advice. The worst that person could do is ignore you or say no.

Networking will take you so much further with your goals than going about achieving them alone. Just remember that no one gets to the top by themselves. There will always be someone out there with more experience or a different outlook who can benefit you in your success. Networking allows you to come in contact with the right people and it will help make the journey into achieving your goals a lot easier.

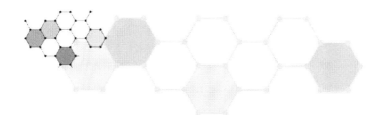

FINDING A GOOD MENTOR

If you are currently a premedical student, there is absolutely no need to pay anyone to help mentor you in your journey to becoming a physician. Mentors can be found for free all around you. There are professors, current medical students, premedical forums on the internet, and a multitude of other free resources.

While I don't knock paid services if you have the money to blow on them, if you're anything like me, then these services can be a huge financial burden. Below are some ways to go about getting the help you need without having to spend too much out-of-pocket.

When it comes to medical school, finding a mentor is not as hard as people like to make it. The Student Doctor Network (SDN) has many forums where you can ask questions and get advice from current medical students, members of admissions committees, and attending physicians. If you're applying to osteopathic schools, the American Osteopathic Association (AOA) went out of its way to make a website dedicated to making physician mentors available to both premedical and medical students alike. This website can be found by searching "AOA iLearn Mentor Program."

A few of my blog readers asked about ways to contact DO's for shadowing opportunities, and I think this would be excellent for that.

As far as I am aware, a program like this does not exist through the Association of American Medical Colleges (AAMC), but finding a physician mentor can be as simple as looking through a local physician directory and making a few phone calls.

You could utilize professors as mentors and contact medical schools that you're interested in and set-up an appointment to discuss the ways in which you can become a more competitive applicant. Once you have found a mentor, they can help guide you through the application process and be a source of encouragement. Many individuals will do this for free, so again, I see no point in paying for this.

Put in the Effort

Basically, this chapter was my way of saying that I do not promote high-cost companies as a resource to premedical students. I was not in a position to afford these companies when I was going through the process, and I do not want my readers to feel that they need to shell out cash in order for their applications to stand out. Even if you do not personally know anyone who can help you with your application, or if you have been out of school a while, all it takes is a little effort to find the help you need. Don't be afraid to reach out of your comfort zone and find the individuals who can help you achieve your goals.

Applying to medical school alone is a very expensive process; Finding the help and support you need shouldn't be.

Making the Decision to Apply

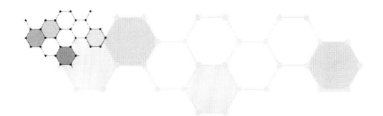

DON'T WAIT ON SUCCESS; MAKE IT HAPPEN!

When Success Happens

When and where do success and achievement always happen? They always happen here and now.

This is the moment when you can choose to either work toward your dreams or to let them fade away. Now is when you take the specific actions that create the reality of your life.

Successful achievement is not some far off, future concept that might happen someday. Achievement is very real, and comes about as a result of what you do now.

You will not ever get anything done if you keep scheduling it for someday. What you do with right now is what truly makes a **difference in your life.**

Your future consequences are determined right here, right now, based on what you do with this day. This is when you can put real life and substance into your dreams.

Delight in this moment and give your very best to it. For in this moment is when you are creating your life, and in this moment is **when success happens.**

Ralph Marston – The Daily Motivator

The above gem was sent to me a few years ago. For those of you who don't know me, I am a HUGE procrastinator! I have so many ideas and a list of things that I want to do in all areas of life, but I always find a way to put them off. For instance, I had the majority of this book completed in July 2016, but now, in July 2019, I am just now starting the editing process and putting it into fruition. It has always been easier for me to say that I will have better luck with something if I wait for the perfect time, but in reality, now is the best time to do anything. Tomorrow is not promised for anyone and I want to live my life with no regrets.

So what does this have to do with medical school?

Well, as a non-traditional student, I know how easy it is to put off things like completing pre-requisites, submitting an application, or taking the MCAT. Life doesn't stop when you apply to or enter medical school, so it's best to just jump right in and do what needs to be done. I often get asked when someone should apply to medical school. Often my readers state they have a future MCAT score pending, have a chance to improve their grades in an upcoming semester, or that they are not sure if their application is truly ready to be submitted. You'll never know if you can be successful at something if you never even begin to do it. Risk-taking is a part of the game, and the results can be pleasantly surprising.

With that being said, both the AMCAS and AACOMAS applications typically open for submissions in June. If you have been putting off applying, but you think you might have a solid chance of being successful, then go for it! If you have been studying for months on end for the MCAT but you want to push the date back because you are nervous that you won't do well, take it anyway. If you don't feel adequately prepared to apply for or take the MCAT, then register for classes, get started on those extracurricular activities, or do whatever you need to succeed. Like the start of this chapter says: success starts now, so what are you waiting for?

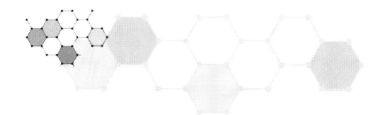

APPLICATION TIMELINE

I am frequently asked about the timing of my application submissions. For the 2013-2014 application cycle, I made sure to apply as soon as the application cycle opened. Everyone's experience may be a little bit different from mine, but I figured it would still be helpful to a few people out there. The below dates are all from memory, and it has been quite a few years since I first applied, so please forgive me if any of the dates are a little bit off.

January/February

If you will be applying for any fee waivers or financial assistance, this is the best time to make sure that you file your taxes and fill out the Free Application for Federal Student Aid (FAFSA). Both MD and DO medical schools will require this. Also, if you plan on taking the MCAT in the spring, this will allow you to apply for the AAMC Fee Assistance Program (FAP) fee waiver as soon as possible. I had already paid for my MCAT by the time I applied for mine, but it would have saved me quite a bit of money had I done it earlier.

May

The AACOMAS application should open around May 1st, and the AMCAS application opens shortly after that. You won't be able to submit the application until June, but it gives you a month to add everything into your application and make sure it's perfect. The sooner you get started the better because once submitted it can take up to six weeks to process. You should also send in your transcripts at this time.

This is also the time when you can submit the AACOMAS fee waiver application. I submitted mine around the first week of May, and I was approved on May 24th. This will allow you to apply to three DO schools for free.

For those of you planning to take the MCAT, this is a good time to do so because it will ensure that you receive your scores back in June or early July. A lot of schools will wait on these scores, so if you have never taken it, the earlier the better. I did not need to worry about taking the MCAT early for my final application cycle because I still had scores that were valid (they're good for three years), so I scheduled mine for July.

Lastly, start asking for letters of recommendation and try to give a one to two-month deadline. Be sure to follow-up with your writers because they tend to have busy lives and can forget. You can also ask for these at the start of the year and store the letters in Interfolio. It is a super convenient secure online storage option and allows you to send your letters to both MD and DO application services.

June

Because I received a fee waiver in advance and started on my application a month prior, I was able to submit my AACOMAS application on the first week that submissions were allowed. I also submitted my AAMC FAP application on June 10th and was approved on June 14th. This allowed me to apply to 14 allopathic schools for free, take the MCAT at reduced cost, get free MCAT assessment tests, and free Medical School Admissions Requirements (MSAR) and Getting to Know the MCAT books. Unfortunately, I had already paid for these items months prior, so it really was of no benefit to me. The reduced MCAT fee did come in handy when I re-took it in September though.

You want to submit as early as possible, but don't stress if you don't get your application in within the first week. The application services do not send the applications to schools until weeks later, so the only benefit is being a part of the first batch of applications that are transmitted.

July

AACOMAS released my application around the fourth of July my final cycle, and I started receiving secondaries the next day. I believe AMCAS had a bit of a delay, so I wasn't verified until August 2nd. Secondary applications came in pretty fast. I made sure to have all secondaries mailed back within two weeks of receiving them. The Student Doctor Network website is a great resource for pre-writing your secondary responses because it provides the prompts given the previous year. These typically do not change, so it helps save some time.

August-September

This time was spent filling out secondary applications and playing the waiting game.

October

I received my interview invite around the 16th of October, but I was first complete at the school around August 27th. It just goes to show how long of a wait it can be sometimes.

November

I had my first interview and emailed an acceptance a few days later. It was my first-choice school, so I was officially done!

December-May

Unfortunately, most people will not get an acceptance so early in the cycle. This is why I recommend you apply as early as possible! Don't feel discouraged if you haven't been given an invite or an acceptance before March because as you can see, there are still five more months to go and this is a very long process.

I have no experience with wait-lists, but I've heard stories of some people not being accepted until a few days before classes started! So, continue to keep the faith and think good thoughts if you have been placed on a wait-list.

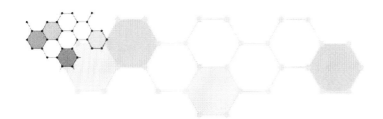

MONEY MATTERS

Looking back at my past checking account made me realize one thing: applying to medical school is a super expensive process! I sent a $250 deposit to hold my seat when I first got my acceptance letter, and later sent a final deposit of $1500.

That's vacation money!

I knew it would all be worth it, so I wasn't too upset. I know quite a few of you will be applying to medical school soon, so I wanted to include this chapter to give you an idea of the expenses you will be incurring during the application process. This way, you can properly budget for everything.

I've split everything below into categories, and I hope it helps. Good luck to all those who will be applying this year!

MCAT:

$315 – $370 (Apparently the test is now in zones. The earlier you register, the cheaper the price)

Letters of Recommendation:

For my LORs, I used Interfolio. It's completely free for your letter writers, but the cost is around $48 per year and it allows for up to 50 academic deliveries. Fortunately, they do not charge you for multiple submissions to the same schools, and this comes in handy when you have to get updated letters because of a lack of signature or letterhead (yes, this did happen to me).

Transcripts:

The school that I attended for undergrad sends transcripts for free, but the other schools on my record had fees of $5-$10, so keep this in mind. You will need to send them to the application services and to the school that you eventually become accepted to.

AACOM application fees:

First school: $195

Each additional school: $45 Secondary Fees: $50 – $200

AMCAS application fees:

First school: $170

Each additional school: $40 Secondary fees: $50-$200 per school

Interviews:

This is really specific to the school and the distance of the school from where you live. This number could easily get into the thousands, so keep that in mind. I won't give the individual costs, but here are the things you should budget for:

Hotel	Food
Rental car	Gas
Flights and baggage fees	Business suit and shoes

Once Accepted:

The fees don't stop after you get accepted, so make sure you budget for the following:

- **Class Deposit** (I'm sure it is a lot more now, but for my medical school in 2014, this was $250 within 30 days and then $1500 before April 1st)

- **Background check fee**

- **Costs for immunizations and physical exam**

- **Moving expenses**

- **One to two months of rent, groceries, and personal expenses while you wait for financial aid to kick in** (typically in the middle of the month when classes start)

- **School supplies**

I believe that's everything, although I may have missed a thing or two. I also want to add that making sure your credit score is top notch will help you out so much when it comes to school. Some loans require a credit check, so it helps to be mindful of maintaining a good credit score and history. It can also come in handy in emergency situations, so stay on the safe side.

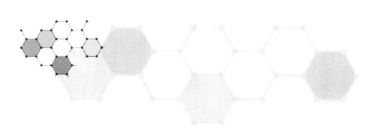

PURSUING OSTEOPATHIC MEDICINE

I attended an osteopathic medical school, and people tend to have a lot of questions about the type of education I received and what it means to be an osteopathic physician. Hopefully, this chapter will provide some good insight.

What is an osteopathic physician and how does this differ from being an MD?

There are only two types of fully licensed physicians in the United States: Osteopathic physicians who bear a D.O. after their name, and allopathic physicians who have an M.D. after their name. For the most part, there really are no differences between the two.

Osteopathic physicians are taught to view medicine in a holistic manner, which means if you come in for a abdominal pain, the general idea is that a DO will look at all areas of an individual's body rather than focusing on the single area of concern. I believe the osteopathic philosophy is to "treat the person and not the symptoms." It is one of the things that I admire most about DO's, and I do feel that it makes for a better physician. This is not to say that MD's don't do the same, but I believe osteopathic medicine places a lot more emphasis on this. DO's also have an added step in their training that consists of OMT (more below), but that is pretty much it for the differences between the two. DO's are not naturopaths or anything else that involves alternative medicine. It is just that a lot of people assume when they go to the doctor they are seeing an MD, and I believe this adds to many misconceptions about DO's. As a premedical student, I didn't like it when some DO's would only refer to themselves as Dr. and leave off the "DO" part of their titles. Now as a practicing physician, I completely understand because it helps ease some of the confusion that patients tend to have. I am always happy to educate individuals regarding the differences, but honestly, there is very little difference between an MD and DO outside of the extra training we receive during medical school.

What is OMT and do all osteopathic physicians use it?

DO's have to learn osteopathic manipulation treatment (OMT) in medical school which is, in a very condensed form of the term, using your hands to diagnose and treat a patient. This is mostly useful for patients who experience chronic pain such as muscle aches and the like. In my opinion, OMT is like combining the skills of a chiropractor with a masseuse.

Not all physicians use OMT though. In my shadowing experiences, I never saw any of my mentors use OMT. My chosen field of practice is surgery, and outside of a few very limited techniques such as colonic stimulation for constipation, it is not something that is used often in this field. Maybe some surgeons find a way to incorporate it beforehand, but I have personally never witnessed it.

Outside of medical school, the only time I ever saw OMT being demonstrated was during medical conferences. As a premedical student, I volunteered to be a dummy for it at a conference, and it worked. A couple of pulls, cracks, and body contorting and I didn't have any shoulder pain for a few weeks after the conference. I also had a lot of back and shoulder pain as a medical student from the long hours of studying, and it was nice having my professors around to manipulate me every now and then. I felt like a new person after every session!

Does an osteopathic physician receive training in a hospital?

Believe it or not, as a premedical student, my boss asked me this question when he first found out where I was accepted. I have no idea where else a physician would be able to receive their clinical training from, so this is just a weird question to me. Like MDs, DOs attend school for four years with two years of classroom training and two years of clinical training. Yes, the clinical training does take place at hospitals and does include hospital rotations just like our MD counterparts. I even rotated with MD medical students during my time in medical school, and now as a physician, I often have MD medical students on my service who I help teach and train.

Is it harder to specialize or gain acceptance as a DO?

As an osteopathic physician, I have found that there are still some obstacles in specializing in competitive fields, but this is mostly due to there still being a few misconceptions about osteopathic medicine. These obstacles are being broken down daily, with the most recent accomplishment being a merger between MD and DO residency programs. I personally know of osteopathic physicians in highly competitive fields such as neurosurgery, dermatology, orthopedic surgery, dermatology, etc., so there is nothing an osteopathic physician cannot achieve. I believe if an individual works hard and achieves high board scores, any field is possible to attain.

As for the acceptance, looking at forums such as the Student Doctor Network, it would appear that there is a strong bias against DO's.

Oddly enough, in my interactions with MDs as a medical student they were all very accepting of DO's and told me that they were happy to work with them. One told me that a doctor is a doctor, and I shouldn't be concerned with the negative stuff that I have read. The DO's that I knew prior to becoming a medical student expressed the same. Most did acknowledge there was a strong bias a long time ago, but this is no longer the case.

Why did I choose DO?

For me, it never really mattered what initials are behind my name. I want to be the best possible physician I can be, and osteopathic medicine offered this to me. As a premedical student, I loved the holistic approach to medicine, and the DO's I did know were highly respected. I also liked that osteopathic medical schools take a holistic approach to viewing their applicants. I am more than just my numbers, and I love that the osteopathic medical schools take this into consideration. I have always been into breaking down barriers and exploring new heights, and osteopathic medicine gave me the opportunity to accomplish this while gaining more recognition for osteopathic physicians. Osteopathic medicine is a profession that I am proud to be a member of, and if I had to go back and choose again, I would not change a thing.

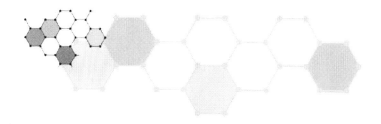

LETTERS OF RECOMMENDATION
(LORs)

It is never too early to start thinking about obtaining letters of recommendation. I've been asked a few questions about this, so this chapter is my attempt to answer them.

When should I ask for letters of recommendation?

I advise you to ask for letters of recommendation two months in advance of when you need them. Usually, LORs aren't needed until you complete the secondary application, which will be around July or August if you submit at the very beginning. Giving two months will allow you to send a monthly or even gentle weekly reminders if your letter still has not been written. It is important to realize that your letter writers most likely lead busy lives, so it will be up to you to make sure the letters get submitted in a timely fashion.

How do I approach and ask potential writers?

If you're still in school, you can always swing by during office hours and ask professors. Just tell them a little about yourself and your goals. Ask them if they would be able to write a "strong" letter of recommendation. Don't be afraid to ask, even if you haven't interacted much with your professors. In the past, professors who did not know me very well usually asked me for a copy of my curriculum vitae (CV, better known as resume) and personal statement to help them write the letter.

If you have taken online classes or have since moved away from school, e-mail is another great idea. I have asked for LORs by e-mail before, and it really has not been a problem. At most, the letter writer will want more information about you, which shouldn't be too hard to provide. I have never been denied a request for a letter, and I really do think people enjoy writing them. Just make sure to give them enough time. These are very busy people!

In the case of physicians, when you initially contact them for shadowing, don't be afraid to ask if they would also be willing to write a good LOR. They may not know enough about you to write a strong letter, but they can definitely give a character reference and their thoughts on how much interest you have shown.

How many LORs should I obtain and who should write them?

At the very minimum, I would say it is good to have at least two letters written by science professors and one from a non-science professor. If you are applying to osteopathic schools, a letter from an osteopathic physician is required or strongly recommended for a lot of schools. It is best to go directly to the websites of the schools that you want to attend and look up the individual requirements.

I remember having one school that specifically only wanted two letters, and another only wanted a letter from the premedical committee. It will save you time if you look up the requirements in advance.

For the 2014 cycle, I had letters from the following:

1. My current boss (non-science/research/work)
2. Science professor from my graduate course (science)
3. Science professor/mentor from undergrad (science/ research)
4. Science professor from graduate course who was also the advisor of my program (science/advisor)
5. Osteopathic physician (DO/clinical)

Should I have my writers send the letters directly to AMCAS or the schools?

The first time I applied to medical school, I had my writers send their letters to each individual school (osteopathic). This can be extremely time-consuming, and it will be hard for you to keep track of everything. I strongly recommend that you set up an Interfolio account (www.interfolio.com). It only costs $48 per year, and you can have your writers send one copy of a letter directly to them. Interfolio will then make copies and send the letters to wherever you designate them to. Your writers will also be able to send in an electronic copy of their letters and digitally sign it on the website. Super convenient! For AMCAS, the letters will need to be sent directly to their letter service, but this can also be done through Interfolio.

As a non-traditional student who has been out of school for a while, what letters should I obtain?

Unfortunately, you will still need to obtain letters from science professors who have previously taught you. It is also good to have LORs from employers and possibly clinical letters from places you may have volunteered. If you completed grad school, also include letters from graduate professors and your advisor.

How important is a letter of recommendation from my school's premedical committee?

For some schools, this letter is very important (and I have the rejections to prove it). As a non-traditional student though, some schools will allow you to substitute science professor letters for this requirement. The premedical committee at my undergraduate institution does not give letters if you have been out of school for more than a few years or if you have a GPA below a 3.0, so unfortunately, I was unable to obtain one. The premedical committee at my graduate school also did not want to write me a letter (based purely on my low undergraduate GPA), and this hurt me at a couple of schools.

Can I pick and choose which letters I want to send to specific schools?

Yes! AMCAS will let you designate which letters you want sent to specific schools. Interfolio is also great for this because you can have all your letters stored in advance and sent to the individual schools (osteopathic only) at your convenience.

How can I check to make sure the letters meet specific requirements?

This is another plug for Interfolio, but they are the absolute best for checking this. I waived all my rights to view my letters, so I had no idea if they met the requirements of being SIGNED and on LETTERHEAD. During my final application cycle, I applied to a medical school that sent me an e-mail stating that some of my letters did not have this. I would not have known otherwise! After that, I made it a point to call Interfolio and ask them which letters did not meet the requirements. The customer service representatives will go through each of your letters and let you know if they have what is needed. You can then send another request to your writers, and they will replace the letters. This is very invaluable because it can mean the difference between an automatic rejection or an interview.

Should I wait to submit my application until I have received all my letters?

As soon as you are ready to submit the application, go ahead and do so. The letters will be required to mark your application as complete once you receive the secondary and submit it. Some schools reject pre-secondary, so there is no need to send letters until you have been asked to do so.

Should I mention osteopathic medicine in my personal statement?

Even if you are only applying to osteopathic medical schools, in my opinion, you should not write about osteopathic medicine in your personal statement. When you receive secondary applications, the majority of them will ask, "why this school?" and "why osteopathic medicine?". If you write about this in your personal statement, you will have a really hard time answering the question in your secondary essays without sounding redundant. The personal statement should focus on your desire to become a physician and seek to answer the question, "why medicine?".

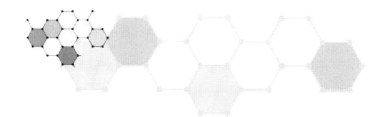

CHOOSING A MEDICAL SCHOOL: APPLY BROADLY!

I cannot stress this enough when it comes to medical school applications: APPLY BROADLY!

The entire process is an extreme crapshoot and there is no such thing as a safety school. You may think you have a great chance at one school only to end up being rejected pre-secondary. The same can apply to schools that you think are a reach. When I applied during my final cycle, I did not think I had even the slightest chance at the school I was accepted to, even though my heart was set on it. I had previously been rejected from the school and various forum boards said they did not take any MCAT section with a score of less than an 8 (based on the old exam scoring system). Obviously, that was not the case, although it may have been more of a general guideline than a set rule. Additionally, there were a few schools that I received secondary applications to that heavily screen the primary applications. I'm pretty sure my graduate school GPA was taken highly into consideration even though it was not explicitly mentioned on their websites. I even received e-mails from some of these schools stating that they were interested in receiving my MCAT scores after a retake to help with their decisions. The fact that I could not increase my score was definitely a factor in some of my rejections.

The point of this section is not to discourage anyone, but to make sure you don't make some of the same mistakes I did in my first two application cycles. A new application cycle opens every year, and I want everyone to have the best possible chance of gaining an acceptance. Applying to medical school is an expensive process, but having to re-apply because you did not choose the right schools the first time can be even more expensive. It is super important to utilize the AACOM Osteopathic Medical College Information Book and AAMC Medical School Admissions Requirements (MSAR) books to pick the right schools for you. The next section will also discuss how I went about selecting some of my schools. If there is that one school that you feel you don't have the slightest chance at, but your heart is set on it, apply anyway. I can say from experience that it just might result in some great news.

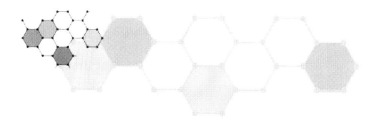

SELECTING SCHOOLS AND NARROWING DOWN THE LIST

Another question I get asked a lot involves the number of schools I applied to and how I made my choices. I really think this is dependent on your individual needs, but I don't mind sharing how I narrowed down my school list.

I've heard that the average applicant will apply to 10-15 schools. I didn't consider myself to be an average applicant in the process, so I applied to 26 schools (both MD and DO). When selecting schools, I considered the following factors:

- **GPA/MCAT:** I looked at the average stats of accepted applicants for all the schools I was interested in. For MD schools, the MSAR is a valuable source for this because it lists all this information and more for every school. It's not free, but if you are planning on applying to any MD school then you absolutely need it. It lists both the top and bottom tenth percentile of GPAs and MCAT scores accepted by each school, along with other very important information. For DO schools, I used the Osteopathic Medical College Information

Book which can be found as a pdf file for free on the AACOM website. It doesn't list the individual accepted GPA and MCAT stats for each school, but it will tell you the minimum GPA needed to obtain a secondary. This helped me avoid applying to schools that would automatically screen me out.

- **Graduate degrees:** I looked at the percentage of matriculants that held a graduate degree. I figured schools with a higher percentage of students with advanced degrees probably considered those grades more heavily than undergraduate grades. This was just a guess on my part and might not be entirely accurate.

- **Race/Ethnicity data:** This was entirely a personal thing, but I avoided applying to some schools that listed the percentage of black applicants as being zero or less than one percent. I really don't mind being the only black person in a class, but having absolutely no black matriculants felt somewhat odd to me.

- **Location:** I know beggars can't be choosers, but I just couldn't see myself living out in the middle of nowhere with absolutely no support system or places I could take my daughter for bonding time. Also, if I was going to be without a close support system, I wanted to at least be in a place with readily accessible babysitters in case of emergencies.

- **Cost:** One school I looked at had the tuition listed at $80,000 a year. Add housing and other costs to that, and it really adds up. I still applied, but had I got accepted, it would have been something to really consider.

- **Mission Statements:** I know this is probably not the most important, but the mission statement of a school will usually tell you if you are a good candidate or not. For example, if a school says that it is committed to training students who will be physicians in a particular area then it might have a regional bias.

- **Regional Bias:** Look closely at the schools' mission statements and in matriculant data for this. Some schools only accept in-state residents. There is no sense in spending your money applying if this doesn't pertain to you. For example, I know of a state with two state medical schools where one only takes in-state residents, and for the other, your parents need to be graduates or you have to have strong and compelling ties to the state.

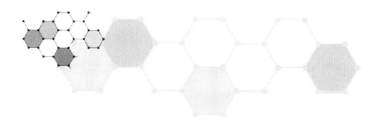

NAILING THE PERSONAL STATEMENT

When it comes to writing personal statements, the advice I hear the most is to answer why medicine and not highlight flaws or any other negative information. It took me a few years to really perfect my personal statement, and I chose to mostly follow my heart when writing it.

The first thing I would say is if you have a low GPA or MCAT score, then absolutely discuss it! While I did not specifically mention any of my low scores, I did bring up the fact that I encountered many obstacles that at times prevented me from doing my best. I went on to mention how these obstacles in retrospect were blessings in disguise, and I highlighted how I benefited from them and grew as an individual. I did not dwell on the negatives, but I did address the fact that I was aware of the issues that may concern admissions committees. It's also important to make sure that your personal statement reflects you and that you are not simply trying to please the individuals reading them. Write about what makes you different from other applicants and discuss what you can bring to the school and the field of medicine in general.

Answering the "Why Medicine?" question was probably the hardest for me. I have literally wanted to be a physician since childhood, and I didn't have the defining moment that so many other people claim to have. I also did not have a compelling story outside of being a single mother. If you do a search for personal statements on the internet, you will quickly find stories of people dealing with family illnesses, going on extraordinary medical mission trips, or having other experiences that really put them on the path to wanting to become a physician. I can't say that this was the case for me. I always had a desire to serve my fellow man, a fascination with the human body, and a pressing need to be a part of something greater than myself. I also had the obvious reasons that I'm sure everyone else applying to medical school has, so I tried to avoid mentioning those in my personal statement.

Another thing that I should add is I did mention being a single mother in my personal statement. It was something that I wrestled with, but one of my mentors made a good point. He said, "If a school does not like the fact that you are a parent, then you should not want to go there anyway." My child is a major part of my life, and to hide that fact would be doing a disservice to both of us. If you are a parent, I think it is important to attend a school that will be able to help you achieve a good balance between your work as a student and your responsibilities as a parent. I'm not saying to only apply to family-friendly schools, but it is good to keep this in mind. There may be times when you will have to miss class due to a sick child or other circumstance, and it would be nice to attend an institution that is willing to work with you.

Make yourself sound awesome, be honest, don't put up a front, and you should be fine. Also, make sure you get multiple people to read your personal statement for you, because they can offer some very valuable advice.

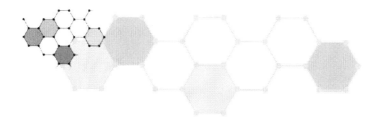

PERSONAL STATEMENT FAQs

This section is an attempt to combine questions I have been frequently asked regarding my personal statement.

Where can I go for help with my personal statement?

One of the greatest resources you can use for help with your personal statement is the forum section of Student Doctor Network. This forum has current medical students, school administration members, and fellow students who are willing to look over, revise, and offer suggestions to improve your personal statement completely FREE OF CHARGE! In my opinion, there is no reason not to take advantage of the resource.

If you are someone who does not want complete strangers to read your personal statement, there are other options as well. If your school does not have a writing center, you could still take your personal statement to any English professor and ask them for help with grammar and such. Also, if you have a physician who you shadow, don't be afraid to ask them for help in looking over your personal statement. They can be one some of the best resources because they know how the game works. I remember having an emergency room appointment a few years back, and randomly asking one of the residents if they would take a look at my personal statement. The person didn't even hesitate to give me their e-mail address, and they provided great feedback after I sent them my personal statement.

How do I include all of my extracurricular activities (ECs) in my personal statement?

There's really no need to write about every extracurricular activity you have ever done in the personal statement. Admissions committees can already view this in your overall application, and it will come off as redundant. If there was a particularly meaningful experience that you had while on a mission trip or volunteering then write about that, but don't try to list all your ECs in paragraph form. Just focus on one aspect. You could even center your whole personal statement over one experience and try to tie in how the other ECs either helped you get to that point or how you discovered new extracurricular activities because of the experience.

How did you talk about your extracurricular activities in your personal statement?

I talked about a few of my ECs in my personal statement, but it was really light. I mentioned them to show how I still continued to be involved even though I had other responsibilities to deal with. I did not mention anything specific. I just mentioned how I took leadership positions within a few organizations, and I wrote briefly about how these organizations gave me the opportunity to stay involved.

Were you specific about osteopathy in your personal statement? I heard some people saying that it's better to be specific in the secondary so that it doesn't sound repetitive. What do you think?

Do not write about osteopathic medicine in your personal statement.

When you receive secondary applications, many of them will ask "why this school" and/or "why osteopathic medicine". If you address it in your personal statement, you will have a really hard time answering the question in your secondary essays. Just write about your desire to be a physician. (Note: make sure you say osteopathic medicine. Some people take offense to the word "osteopathy" because it can mean something entirely different overseas).

How long was your personal statement? (# of words)

For AMCAS, my personal statement was 869 words and came out to be 4693 characters with spaces. The max character limit for AMCAS is 5300.

For AACOMAS, my personal statement was 790 words and 4485 characters with spaces according to Microsoft Word. On my application, it was calculated as a total of 4500 characters which is the max limit for the AACOMAS application.

Where can I find examples of personal statements and meaningful experience essays?

Finding good personal statement examples was one of the hardest things for me when I originally drafted my personal statement. This was over 10 years ago, but now examples are luckily only a short click away. Below are two really good resources I previously found, and you can find my own complete personal statement in the next section:

Medical School Essays that Made a Difference by **The Princeton Review** – This was literally the only thing I used for examples when I originally drafted my personal statement. It helped me formulate a good starting point, but I felt that my first essay was too cookie-cutter because of it. To correct this, I dramatically changed my personal statement over the years to reflect me and my growth. Unfortunately, this book isn't available online.

http://www.accepted.com/medical/sampleessays.aspx – Good example personal statements from Accepted.com

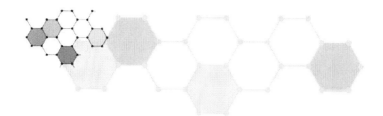

MY FULL PERSONAL STATEMENT

I hope this can help those of you who are looking for an example of a personal statement. I often get asked many questions about what I included in my personal statement, so hopefully this will answer them. Just remember that not every personal statement will look like this, and everyone should have a different and unique story to tell. This personal statement is a result from years of corrections, and I made sure to have multiple people read it and give me their input. Also, a lot of people told me to remove the first sentence, but I felt it described me perfectly, so I left it in. This is the personal statement I used for my AACOMAS application, and the one I used for AMCAS only differed by having an additional sentence or two.

I am sharing this one since my acceptance was to an osteopathic school. **It should go without saying, but my personal statement should not be copied or used as your own.** What I have written below is a representation of me, and only personal to me. Please find experiences that represent you well and give an accurate reflection of why you are pursuing medicine when you go write your own personal statement. Enjoy!

****

I wish I could say that my academic performance was the result of partying or carelessness, but the truth is that I put a lot of blood, sweat, and tears into my education. My desire to pursue medicine stems from my goal of wanting to help those in need and put others before myself, and becoming a physician would allow me to continue to do so while improving lives in the process. There have been many obstacles in trying to achieve this goal, but in retrospect, these hurdles not only motivated me more towards my ambitions, but they fueled my desire to really explore the field of medicine. I also learned to find the positives out of every situation and not let my past dictate my future. It is because of this that I feel I am an excellent candidate for medical school, and that no matter what challenges or obstacles may be presented, I will find a way to achieve my goal of becoming a physician.

My undergraduate years were both rewarding and demanding due to the fact that I became a mother, a wife, went through a divorce, and had to find a balance between school and family issues, all while working to make ends meet. My first semester at LSU was met with Hurricane Katrina, which led to class cancellations and caused the institution to become an emergency center for some of the victims. This was my first time experiencing a natural disaster of this magnitude, and I volunteered my time by helping with patient registration, triage, donation sorting, and by trying to console those who had lost everything in the storm. It was at this point where I learned that compassion and understanding can sometimes do more for a person than just trying to treat them, and this experience really amplified my desire to pursue medicine and dedicate my time and resources to all those in need in and around my community.

I gave birth to my daughter during the fall semester of my sophomore year, and while this halted my ability to donate all of my time and energy to volunteering, the maturing challenges presented with raising a child far outshined the negatives. While adjusting to motherhood, I was still able to persevere and continue to pursue my interest in medicine by physician shadowing and becoming involved in various medically-related organizations.

Shadowing was an especially positive experience because I was able to physically see if medicine was the right choice for me, and it allowed me to develop a more solid understanding of what it takes to become a physician.

I took leadership positions in a few organizations, and helped others become more involved as well. These positions provided unique opportunities to help the community which ranged from painting houses for the elderly to spreading HIV/AIDS awareness to the public. I also found meaningful employment in places where I was able to continue to give back to the community, which included everything from teaching autistic children to working for the Battered Women's Program. Right now, I am fully involved in research, and I volunteer weekly at my local hospital. I am also in a graduate program working to further enhance my academic skills. Being able to use my experiences to make a change for the better and impact lives helped shaped me into the person I am today, and I am thankful for it. I feel that a great sense of humility and a deep drive has been instilled in me, and because of this, I know that I have something meaningful to bring to the field of medicine.

I am proof that it is possible to overcome circumstances, and by achieving my dream of becoming a physician, I hope to push others to accomplish their goals as well. Along with my innate desire to help others, I have a strong interest in the human body and in solving complex problems, and I want to be able to help a person medically from all aspects, including being involved in both the diagnosis and treatment of patients. Furthermore, medicine would not only give me a lifelong learning experience, but it would allow me to essentially dedicate myself to a lifetime of service. I truly feel that medicine is my calling in life, and although there may be many obstacles along the way, I refuse to give up on my dream. At the 2008 SNMA medical conference, Dr. Barbara Ross-Lee stated that qualifications are a measure of opportunity and not of worth, and I am grateful for the chance to finally be able to show my true worth in my journey to becoming a physician and beyond.

Thank you for your time and interest in my application.

****

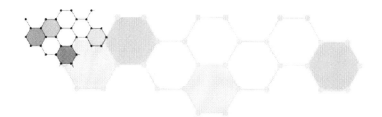

INTERVIEW DAY BASICS

For a lot of people, preparing for the interview is one of the most stressful parts of the application process. There are concerns about what to wear, what questions will be asked, suitable hotels, the decision to fly or drive, how early to arrive and the list goes on. Below I will detail my medical school interview experience and try to give a little advice along the way.

Receiving an interview invite

I was so excited when I received my first interview invitation. I had just made it to work one morning and was getting out of my car when I heard the e-mail notification go off on my phone. I had a separate e-mail address and sound for medical schools, so I figured it was another rejection e-mail and braced myself for the worse. I could have screamed when I saw that it was the exact opposite! This was in early October, but the invitation was for December. I wasn't too concerned at first because I figured it would give me enough time to prepare.

I logged onto the Student Doctor Network (SDN) forum to share the news with others in the school-specific section, and I noticed that many people were getting invites at the same school with much earlier dates. As the weeks went on this started to worry me, plus I had a final exam in my on-campus class the day after my original interview date, so I decided to call the school. I figured they had given me a late invitation since I was out of state, so when I called I let the school know I had no problem making it from out of state, and if an earlier interview slot opened I would be happy to take it.

This was on a Friday afternoon, and to my surprise the person in admissions replied with "Can you be here Monday?" I was ecstatic and immediately said yes! And so my interview preparation began....

Attire

The first thing I needed to decide was what I would wear to the interview. Fortunately, I attended quite a few conferences and had a closet full of professional attire. Many people said that a dress suit is best for females, but I just couldn't bring myself to go out and buy one. I feel confident in a pant suit and I am always cold, so the more covered the better. I did go out and buy a blouse that completely covered my chest, and I wore this underneath my suit jacket. I also went and bought lower heels. I love my 4, 5, and 6 inch heels, but sadly they are not appropriate for interviews. Overall, I was very happy with my choice. The heels were very comfortable for walking during the tour, and I did not have to worry about being self-conscious over skirt length. It also seemed that everyone in the interview group wore dark colors, so it was a good way to fit in.

Getting There

The school where I interviewed and attended was 8 hours away from where I lived at the time. I thought about flying, but would have had to get a rental car once in the area. Also, with the new interview date only two days away, plane prices were ridiculous. Driving was cheaper and gave me some much-needed time to myself, so this was a no-brainer for me.

Lodging

The school's website mentioned that hotels in the area gave discounts to visiting people, so I called up one and was able to get a rate of $75/night. I was only staying one night, and they offered late check-out for free. Plus, it was only 1 mile away from the school which meant less stress for me in the morning.

The Day Before / Preparation

Most of the Sunday before my interview was spent driving. Once I made it to the hotel, I checked in and then decided to find the school. I'm glad I did this. The GPS I was using had not been updated so it got me a little bit lost. I was so thankful that my phone had navigation (now pretty much common for everyone), and it literally only took 2 minutes to make it to the school and back. There was a restaurant directly across the street from the hotel, so I took the time to order some take-out, and went back to my room to go over stuff for my interview.

For my interview, I utilized a ton of resources. I think the best one is the interview section on the SDN forums. It has all the questions that were asked to previous interviewees, along with their thoughts on each school and what to expect. I also found a list on the internet from a premedical committee with at least 100 questions that could be asked. I went over every single question and thought about what my responses would be. I even looked into recent health issues in the news and prepared myself with questions that could be asked from that. I even made out a list of about 20 questions to ask during my interview just in case I forgot later on. I did all this for about 2 hours while eating my take-out and watching an award show that night. I made sure I went to sleep by midnight so that I could be well-rested.

The Big Day

The day of my interview I woke up around 6:45 for an 8am interview. I was showered, dressed, and out the door by 7:40. I made it to the school around 7:45, and we all signed in, got our name tags, and waited until around 8 or 8:15 (I can't quite remember). We were then met by a person from admissions who spoke to us and gave us folders with financial aid and other school information. After this was done, we were taken into a computer room where we had 30 minutes to type out our responses to a few pre-interview questions. I really liked this because it gave me time to really think about what I wanted to say, and it further prepared me for my interview. From there, our group was given a complete tour of the school by one of the student ambassadors. Afterwards, we were taken into a room where there were current students and other people from admissions. This is where we found out who our interviewers were, and we waited while each student took their turn. There was food, and everyone in the room was more than happy to answer all of our questions about the school. The admissions team really did an excellent job making us feel more comfortable and easing our nerves that morning.

When it came my turn to interview, I was taken into a room and my interviewers were a faculty member and medical student. My interview was extremely laid back and the questions were mostly designed to get to know me as a person. I was prepared to answer any questions about my shortcomings, but I was asked nothing about my grades or scores. Most of the questions were geared towards my study habits, why I chose that particular school, and what I liked to do in my spare time. This made me really happy. They also didn't mind the million questions I had, and I appreciated that there was a student interviewing me as well because some of my questions were centered on student life.

After the interview, I was done for the day. I made it back to my hotel around 11:30 and I was back on the road home by 12. I had promised my daughter I would be home to tuck her in that night and I made it back with five minutes to spare.

Final Thoughts

The best thing I could say about the interview is to be yourself. I asked a lot of questions and even made sure that I spoke with current students. Medical school is a place where you will be spending the majority of your time for the next four years, so make sure that you absolutely love it. I made note of how helpful the admissions team was, how happy the students were, and I asked the important questions about attendance, tests, and all that other good stuff. I left feeling really good about both the school and my interview, and this feeling was magnified when I received the acceptance e-mail four days later.

.

DEALING WITH REJECTION

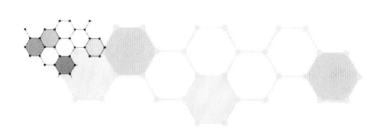

MY PERSONAL STORY OF REJECTION: WHY IT'S NOT THE END OF THE ROAD

Before my medical school acceptance, I previously applied to the same school during the 2008-2009 application cycle. I was initially rejected but kept the original rejection letter. For me, rejection never meant that my journey was over or that I had failed. In my eyes, the only failure in life is giving up too soon. Because it was my first-choice school, I held onto my rejection letter with the thought in mind that I would frame it one day when my acceptance letter came. It took over four years for the acceptance to come, but it finally happened. The rejection only added fuel to my fire and made me even more determined. I still hold onto both my rejection and acceptance letters, and it served as a source of inspiration that helped push me through medical school.

I've seen a lot of people get rejected one time and decide to give up. Things may not always happen the way you want them to or when you want them to, but you have to have faith that everything will fall into place when the time is right. Looking back now, getting a rejection was one of the best things that could have ever happened to me. It allowed me to grow as an individual and experience more of what life has to offer. Also, I do not know how I would have managed to raise a toddler and handle medical school at the same time with no support system in place. They say that hindsight is 20/20, and I'm really beginning to understand that now. I'm rooting for all my readers to get accepted on the first try, but if that doesn't happen, I hope reading this will inspire you to not give up.

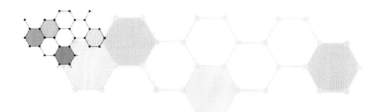

BECOMING A REAPPLICANT

After 3 application cycles, I cannot stress enough how good it felt to finally have an acceptance into medical school! I first applied in 2008, and you could definitely see the growth in my applications. The first time I applied, I could not afford to apply to many schools, and I was lucky enough to receive an AACOMAS fee waiver. This allows for an individual to apply to three osteopathic schools for free, so I picked my three very carefully and hoped for the best. I have no idea what I was thinking applying at the time though because there was nothing notable about my application. While I did have shadowing experience and a letter of recommendation from an osteopathic physician, I had very little extracurricular activities, research, or volunteering experiences mentioned in my application. I think I may have even mentioned job experiences and extracurricular activities from high school. On top of that, my MCAT score was only a 21 and I had a GPA that was below a 2.5. I received rejections from all three schools around May of that year, but due to not passing a biochemistry class that was only offered once a year and having to extend my graduation date, I would not have been able to attend anyway. Needless to say, I was still very upset and not quite sure about my future.

After graduating college in the fall of 2009, I took a job working full-time in a somewhat medically-related research field and I worked on building my resume. By the time 2011 came around, I felt I was ready to re-apply to medical school. This time, I applied to three allopathic schools and they were all attached to Historically Black Colleges and Universities (HBCUs). I re-took the MCAT, but my score literally only increased by one point. I think the only noteworthy thing about my application was that I included all of my experiences, and I completely re-vamped my personal statement to really reflect me. Unfortunately, I was rejected that cycle without any interviews.

Looking back, I can say that my main problems during the cycle were the fact that I definitely did not apply broadly, I took the August MCAT, I applied somewhat late, and I still had not proved to schools that I could handle a heavy course load and succeed.

Fast-forward to 2013, and this time I was going all in. On top of all the extracurricular activities noted from my previous years, I also upped my shadowing experiences, started volunteering every week at my local hospital, and now had research publications under my belt.

By the grace of God, I was accepted into a graduate program in the summer of 2012, and I was doing better than I had ever done in my academic career. This was a risk in itself because graduate courses are not considered in the same fashion as post baccalaureate classes, but I wanted an extra degree to fall back on just in case the application cycle did not work out as well. My graduate classes were not easy, and I think taking classes like chemical thermodynamics, pharmacology, and toxicology really raised some heads. I re-took the MCAT twice that year (yes, that makes a total of four times), but my scores still remained low with a 20 and then a 21. I also applied very broadly within two weeks of the application cycle opening, and I submitted all of my secondary applications within two weeks of receiving them. During my final application cycle, I applied to 26 schools total, and these included both allopathic and osteopathic schools. As of a few months before my matriculation to medical school, I had 1 acceptance, 2 holds, 13 rejections (plus 2 never sent a secondary), I withdrew from two, and I was complete at the others and waiting. I interviewed and was accepted to my first-choice school, so I could confidently and happily say that the application cycle was over for me.

I am living proof that anything is possible despite any shortcomings you may think you have. My advice to any re-applicants is to not give up and to continue to keep pushing for what you want. If you cannot see yourself doing anything else in life, don't be afraid to take risks and go for it. You'll be happy you did.

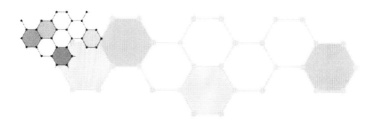

LEARNING FROM REJECTION
/THE NEXT STEPS

Getting rejected is hard, but it can also be an important learning experience. If the application cycle has not ended, try to remain positive. Many schools review applications up until March, and if you are currently on hold or waitlisted, there is still a chance you could gain an acceptance up until the first day of classes. If the application cycle has ended, and there is no chance of you gaining an acceptance, then you will want to start looking at the next steps and how you can prepare to be a better applicant in the future.

The first step is to take a deep breath and realize that this is not the end of the road. Being rejected is tough and can make you feel like medicine is not the right path for you. Try not to fall into this trap. If medicine is meant for you, then it will eventually come, even if it does not happen during the timeline you had envisioned. It is okay to take a moment to deal with your disappointment, but it is important to not wallow in self-pity for too long.

The next step after facing a rejection is finding out what faults were found in your application and/or what you can do to improve with your application. After the application cycle has closed, it is often possible to get in touch with medical school admissions department representatives at the different schools you applied to. They can offer insight into possible red flags they noticed on your application, things you might have been lacking in, or ways that you can improve your application. Not all medical schools will do this, especially during extremely busy times of the year, but it is worth giving it a shot and reaching out to these individuals.

If you notice you are lacking in some areas, then the time after a rejection is a good time to focus on these deficiencies. Since applying to medical school tends to be a year-long process, you will have ample time for improvement, and you can send updates along the way. If your MCAT score is getting in the way, be prepared to schedule a new exam, but make sure you have ample time to study and really focus on your weaknesses. Overall, learn from your rejection so you can be a much stronger applicant the next time around.

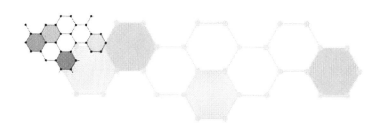

DEALING WITH ADVICE

"Don't base decisions on the advice of those who do not have to deal with the results."

Unknown

So many people love to give advice, but they don't always have your best interests in mind when they do. Just because a particular path worked for one person, does not mean that it will work out the same for you. I think a lot of people may have good intentions when they give advice, but they fail to take into account your situation and the resources you have available. It's easy to come across people who are willing to tell you what you need to do to make it to a particular place, but they have never actually made it there themselves. I've seen this a lot on premedical forums where students who have not yet even been accepted into medical school tend to give the most advice on what you need to do to succeed. My suggestion is to take all advice with a grain of salt and do whatever works best for your situation. Do what works best for you because in the end, you are the only one who has to deal with the consequences of your actions.

THE INSPIRATION
SECTION

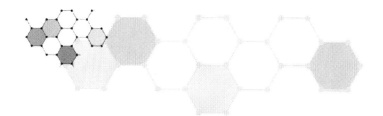

ARE YOU INTERESTED OR COMMITTED?

"There's a difference between interest and commitment. When you're interested in something, you do it only when it's convenient. When you're committed to something, you accept no excuses; only results."

Kenneth H. Blanchard

In my opinion, anyone interested in becoming a physician should realize that medicine is a commitment and not just an interest. An interest is something you explore and get a feel for, but when the going gets tough there is always a back-up plan or a way to drop out. If you are truly committed to something, there is no backing out. That means pushing through some difficult courses, jumping through necessary hoops in the admissions process, dealing with rejection, and even navigating the path alone.

Most physicians (myself included) will tell you that if you can see yourself doing anything else, then do that instead. I have had a chance to explore many interests, and I cannot see myself doing anything else in life. I was committed to becoming a physician, and I will keep reaching for my goals even if that means enduring additional stress, more obstacles, and years of hard work. I know it will all be worth it in the end, but I am not naïve to the fact that it will not be easy getting to that point. There is no Plan B for me, and I am not willing to let anyone talk me out of my dreams. Even when faced with failure and rejection, I do not sit and make excuses. I take responsibility for my shortcomings and work to fix them in order to make myself better.

This section may come off as a bit of a rant, but it really amazes me how easily some people can give up on their goals. Committing to anything in life requires a ton of effort, and nothing good ever comes easy. I've also noticed that some of these same individuals are quick to blame others or a lack of handouts for their shortcomings. Realize that YOU are the only person who can achieve YOUR dreams and do whatever it takes to fulfill that commitment to yourself. The end results will be that much more worth it.

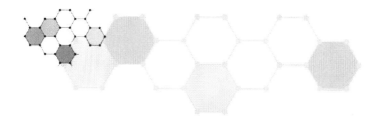

DON'T RUSH

"Good things take time."

I have probably been told the above quote a million times over the years, but I am just now starting to fully understand it. There is absolutely no need to rush to achieve your goals. What is meant to be will be. Frequently I am contacted by individuals looking for the fast-track to becoming a physician without going through all the steps. As someone who completed medical school as an older non-traditional student, I can now look back and appreciate the extra time it has taken me to get to this point. I understand there may be certain circumstances that make you want to push harder so you can move past the difficulties of your current situations, but you should focus on the bigger picture of things. It can be discouraging if things do not work out as planned, but these are the times when you should recoup, reflect, and rejoice in any small new accomplishments that you have made. Do not look at what everyone else around you is doing, but focus on achieving your goals in a way that will benefit you the most in the long run. The summer prior to my medical school acceptance when I was stressing out over having to retake the MCAT, someone told me it was a small thing to worry about, because five years from now it would not matter in the grand scheme of things. At the time, I thought it was a huge deal because most schools wanted me to have a higher score than what I had been able to obtain. After my acceptance, I realized I probably did not need to do the retakes the year prior (I ended up with lower scores), and I now see how the exam was only a small factor in my success. It is now over five years later, and I can tell you that as a physician, no one (patients, colleagues, etc.) cares about how well I did on the MCAT. I could not see it then, but I definitely see it now. So, in a nutshell, don't rush to achieve your goals and try to enjoy yourself in the process.

The following says it best: "Don't miss out on the journey by rushing to get to the destination."

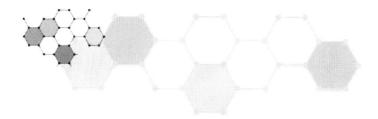

NEVER GIVE UP!

"Never quit. Never give up."

Gabby Douglas

Another question I am asked a lot is why I choose to not settle or give up on my dreams of becoming a physician. Oddly, this is a question I never really thought about, so it was hard for me to come up with an answer at first. The answer is quite simple though. For me, quitting has never been an option, nor will it ever be. I've never allowed myself to have the mindset that I could completely fail because that would have caused me to possibly pursue other options. That's not saying that I haven't failed, but when failure did happen, I looked at other ways of making it work out rather than deciding to quit.

Personally, I think it's all about attitude. If you have the attitude that you are going to be a winner, then eventually one day you will be one. It may not happen when you expect it to, but you need to trust the process. What may seem like failure is in reality an opportunity to define your weaknesses and work on improving yourself.

It's normal for the idea of quitting to cross your mind, but you should realize there are consequences that will come with defeat. I never settled because settling to me is equal to death. I haven't worked for this hard, this long, and survived through everything I have just to quit. My aim is to live a purposeful life and giving up and going through the motions does not accomplish this. I have noticed that usually when people give up, they are so close to winning, and I do not want this to be me. With that being said, whenever I start to feel defeated I just remember that it is always darkest before the light, and that is what keeps me going.

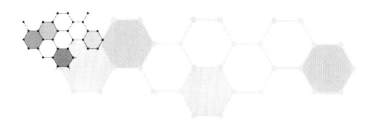

BE POSITIVE!

"Stay Positive. Stay fighting. Stay Brave. Stay ambitious. Stay focused. Stay strong…mentality is everything"

The above conveys what I was trying to say in my last section perfectly! Some people tend to focus on failing before they even begin to accomplish the task. I base this off of visiting premedical forums and seeing the number of posts asking questions about what it takes to be kicked out of school, what will happen if you fail the board exams, etc. Before I began my medical school career, I thought it was crazy to focus on all the negatives before even beginning. I understand it is important to hope for the best and plan for the worst, but thinking you will fail going into anything will only add to your anxiety and increase your chances of doing so. Please do not set yourself up for failure by believing that it will happen before you have even begun.

I will admit that I was just as nervous as everyone else about starting medical school in the fall, but my focus going in was on how I could be the best student possible. In college, I remember how at the beginning of the semester I would calculate the lowest possible grades I could get in order to pass a class with at least a C. If I would do poorly on an exam, I would not be too upset as long as

I could still get enough points on subsequent exams to pass. This mindset allowed me to pass, but that is pretty much all it did. In graduate school, I changed my tune and calculated the amount of points I could miss and still make an A in a class. This not only pushed me to work harder, but it showed me how much more I was capable of doing. I believed I was capable of doing great in every class, and the end results proved this to be true. I went into medical school believing I could be great and fighting for this belief paid off in the end.

I guess the point of all this was just to say stay positive and believe in yourself. Avoid negativity, whether it be from outside individuals or yourself, and keep your eyes on the prize. Maintain a positive mentality and you'll be surprised at how far it can take you.

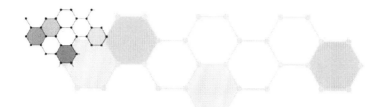

KEEP PUSHING!

"Do not let anyone tell you that you cannot do something. If you have a dream, live it. If you have a desire, act on it. If you have an itch, scratch it. No matter what people tell you, do not let them stop you from living out your dreams. When someone tells you that you cannot do something, go ahead and prove them completely wrong."

Will Smith in "The Pursuit of Happyness"

The above is one of my absolute favorite quotes. A lot of times it can feel like no one supports your dreams and that they are trying to talk you out of pursuing your goals. If something is truly in your heart, you have to learn to ignore the naysayers and continue on your path.

When everything is all said and done, the only thing that will matter is your happiness and that you achieved your goals. Remember misery loves company, and a person saying you cannot accomplish something is probably someone who either failed and gave up or someone who is too afraid to do what you are working on achieving.

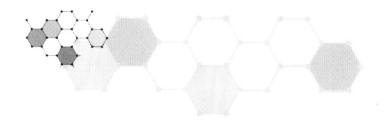

PERSISTENCE IS KEY

Nothing in this world can take the place of persistence. Talent will not: nothing is more common than unsuccessful men with talent. Genius will not; unrewarded genius is almost a proverb. Education will not: the world is full of educated derelicts. Persistence and determination alone are omnipotent.

Calvin Coolidge

Someone sent me the above quote after my fourth MCAT attempt and it really offered some perspective and helped me feel better about my situation. It's easy to get discouraged by the whole application process and want to give up. The funny thing is that one week before I was given an interview invite, I was starting to doubt myself and thought maybe I should give up. It seemed that every time the notification went off on my phone it was yet another rejection e-mail. I had just received back the MCAT scores from my fourth attempt, and I had a Skype interview the same day with the premed committee of my graduate school. They decided in the interview that despite having a high graduate GPA, my low MCAT scores and undergraduate GPA would prevent them from writing me a premedical committee letter of recommendation. This basically meant I would be automatically rejected from the few schools I applied to that absolutely required this. The year 2013 marked over five years of applying to medical school and doing things to make myself a more competitive candidate, and I was just tired!!!! Fortunately, I just could not see myself doing anything else in life (and trust me I've done a lot). The above quote reminds me to this day that nothing in life comes easy. You will face plenty of rejection, and the path will not always be straight-forward, or work out exactly as planned, but these are the things that add character and truly test an individual's ability to succeed. It will all be worth it in the end.

ACCEPTED!
NOW WHAT?!

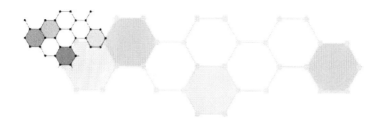

FIRST STEP: CELEBRATE!

You have put in the work, went through the interview process, and you finally receive the coveted medical school acceptance letter. CONGRATULATIONS! Whether you received one acceptance or many, this is a time for celebration. Not only have you proven to a medical school admissions committee that you have what it takes to become a physician, but you no longer have to worry about having to take the dreadful MCAT or dealing with the many hoops you most likely had to jump through to gain an acceptance.

You are about to enter into four years of extremely hard work, many sacrifices, and very little time to take vacations, have long bouts of fun, or pursue outside interests. Take this time to celebrate and get anything out of your system that can interfere with your studies once you begin medical school.

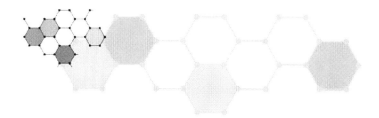

CREATING A "BEFORE MEDICAL SCHOOL BUCKET LIST"

One benefit of being a non-traditional student is I had a lot of time to explore my interests and do some really fun and interesting things prior to starting medical school. From traveling and trying new crazy things to having more time to spend with my daughter, life before medical school was an awesome experience. With that being said, in the months leading up to starting medical school, there were still quite a few things I wanted to accomplish, so I put together a list shortly after my acceptance. Below are a few of my must-do items I crossed off my list prior to assuming the role of becoming a super busy student again.

1. **Go skydiving** ✔
2. **Go ice skating** ✔
3. **Take a vacation (preferably international)** ✔
4. **Start my own blog** ✔
5. **Work on my conversational Spanish** ✔
6. **Chaperone one of my daughter's field trips** ✔
7. **Attend a major live concert (it was the**

Beyoncé and Jay-Z "On the Run" tour) ✔

8. Get my fill of daiquiris ✔

9. Spend a day with my daughter at New Orleans City Park ✔

10. Get a Zulu parade coconut (is it obvious I lived in Louisiana? LOL) ✔

11. Get caught up on all my favorite TV shows ✔

12. Take my daughter to the Georgia Aquarium ✔

13. Try at least 3 New Orleans restaurants that I have not been to ✔

14. Spend one last night partying on Bourbon St (even though I tend to avoid it like the plague LOL) ✔

15. Read at least five books

The biggest thing on my list was taking a vacation, and I was so happy to be able to accomplish the task with a solo trip to Mexico. When I came back from my trip, I was still in party mode, so I headed down to Bourbon Street in New Orleans, danced the night away, and then ended up at Café Du Monde at almost five in the morning eating beignets.

My daughter was in her early childhood years prior to the start of my medical school career, so it was a big deal for me to chaperone one of her field trips. I'm happy that I got to experience that with her, and hopefully she'll keep the memory with her for a long time.

Now you don't have to make a list similar to mine, but I

suggest coming up with a few things that you have been wanting to try. Medical school requires a lot of time, and during the moments when I was stuck in a study hole, it helped to have fun experiences to look back on. The hardest part of medical school is getting accepted, so take the time to celebrate, explore new things, and enjoy yourself.

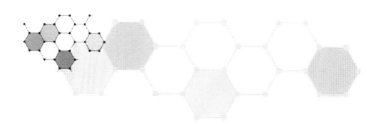

BUDGETING/PAYING FOR MEDICAL SCHOOL

Attending medical school is expensive! Sure there are public medical schools where the tuition can range from $10-20K per year, but if you are not lucky enough to obtain an acceptance or be a resident of the states where these schools are located, you'll be embarking on a very expensive journey. Most medical schools have tuition in the range of $25-50K, but there are quite a few that have tuition prices considerably way higher than this. When I was applying during my final cycle, I encountered a school where the tuition alone was over $80,000! It is very important to be aware of the financial commitment that you will be making prior to entering medical school.

One of the most common questions I used to get asked when people found out I would be attending medical school was how I was going to pay for it. My response: loans, loans, and more loans! I did not come from a family that can afford to help pay for my medical education, and as a single parent, I had the added expense of caring for a young child. I did not plan on working while I am in medical school (which in hindsight would have been impossible), because working throughout my undergraduate years took away from time that I could have been focusing on my education. This was literally my last shot to achieve my dreams, and I did not want anything to get in the way of it. I was "all in" when it came to being a medical student.

So, to answer the question of paying for medical school, I took out subsidized and unsubsidized Stafford loans, along with GradPlus loans to cover the rest. All of my loans were federal loans, and I like to encourage everyone to avoid private loans at all costs! (I took out a few as an undergraduate, and I am still dealing with the headache of having them.) I also applied for a few scholarships and was approved for some with the highest being $5000, and every little bit helped.

Most schools factor in a "cost of living" that will allow you to take out loans for room and board, supplies, transportation, etc. Once my loans took care of tuition and school costs, I received a refund each term used to cover my living expenses. This meant I had to carefully budget each term for around three months at a time, but for me, the amount was more than doable. If you are a fellow non-traditional student with a large family, you will have to take into account what your living expenses will be and contact the school to see if they can increase your cost of living.

Don't Forget the FAFSA

This is a good spot to remind everyone to take some time out to fill out the Free Application for Federal Student Aid (FAFSA). This is the application that will qualify you for student loans and grants once you start medical school. Even if you are not enrolled in school, and do not currently hold an acceptance, still go ahead and fill it out with the codes of the schools that you hope to attend. It can only help you in the long run, and if you do not attend school in the fall there will be no consequences to having filled it out.

Also, check with the schools you plan on attending for individual FAFSA requirements. Even if you are married, an older student, or have children, some schools may still require your parents' information for aid consideration. I believe the majority of allopathic schools have this requirement, but some osteopathic schools will allow you to leave out parent information if you are over a certain age.

The application is really easy and only takes about 10-15 minutes to complete. It's easier if you have already filed your taxes, because you can transport the information directly from the IRS into your application. The link can be easily found by typing "FAFSA" into your search engines.

Apply for Scholarships

Scholarships tend to be something a large number of students overlook. A quick internet search will show thousands of available scholarships that simply require an essay to be written. The number of available scholarships will increase as you progress through your training as a medical student, but there are a few out there for entering medical students. Many students feel they do not have the time to apply for scholarships, but the effort required is very little compared to the amount given. Also, do not be afraid to apply for scholarships with low amounts. You might think that five hundred dollars is nothing compared to the immense amount of tuition you will be paying from medical school, but believe me, every little bit counts. Additionally, make sure to check with the school you will be attending to see if they offer any internal scholarships to incoming students. Many schools do and this can help a lot. Medical school is expensive, but there are ways to make it work. It can be stressful thinking about the many loans you might have to pay back in the future, but paying them off within a reasonable time is possible.

Consider medical school tuition an investment into your future and focus on the moment. Lastly, do not take out more in loans than what is necessary and be smart about your expenses.

If you really want to become a physician, do not be discouraged by the price. Federal loans are readily available, and if you're willing to write a few essays, there are scholarships as well. Thinking about repaying loans can be overwhelming, but there are a ton of programs available to help you pay down your loans when you graduate and there are even some that offer loan forgiveness.

Everyone who I spoke with prior to medical school assured me that paying off medical school loans is possible within ten years, but it may require frugal living for a while. If you're like me, then medical school will probably be the biggest investment that you ever make in life, so I hope this section will help make the decision a little bit easier.

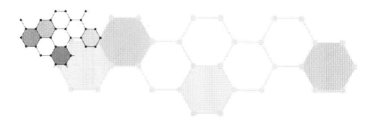

GETTING PREPARED FOR CHANGE

Starting medical school will most likely be a drastic change from your current daily life. I remember leaving a job with a set yearly salary and benefits to basically become a broke student again, and yet I was extremely happy about this. As much as I loved research, I really did (and still do) feel that medicine is my calling and I was ready to pursue the next chapter of my life.

If you are anything like me, an acceptance will also mean that you will be relocating to a place you may or may not be familiar with. You may have to deal with finding a place to live and new schools for your children if you have them. It can be a difficult time but remember to keep in mind that change is usually a good thing. It allows for growth, new opportunities, and a better outlook on life. It can be a lot to take in at first, but a little preparation will go a long way into making the transition smoother.

Whether this is your first-time applying to medical school or you are getting ready to start medical school as a non-traditional student, change is inevitable. Embrace the change. Celebrate the fact that you are pursuing something that will not only positively enhance your life, but the lives of those around you. Remember to take it all one day at a time, and when you finally do accomplish your dreams, do not forget the struggles you faced or the people who helped you get to the place you strived to be. I wish everyone reading this the best of success on their journeys, and I hope this book helps you on the path toward achieving your goals.

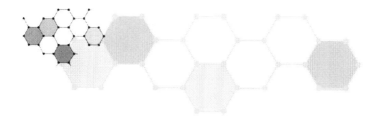

ACKNOWLEDGEMENTS

First things first, I give all thanks, honor, and glory to God for everything I am, for all that I will be, and for everything I have accomplished (past, present, and future).

Thank you to all the aspiring pre-medical students, medical students, and physicians who read my blog and social media posts, email me with questions and comments, and inspire me with your success stories. This book would not be possible without all the support and encouragement you have given me throughout the years.

Tiana, thank you for being the best daughter ever and for giving me the opportunity to grow and learn as your mother. Your patience with me does not go unnoticed, and I am proud of the young woman you are becoming. I love you so much, and I will always be there to support any and all of your dreams. Thank you to Theresa for all you do and the sacrifices you have made to help me fulfill my dreams. I am truly blessed to call you my sister, and thankful that Tiana has you as an aunty, daily role model, friend, and confidant. To all my other brothers and sisters (there's way too many of y'all to name), I thank you for all your love, putting up with me, and not getting upset when I don't keep in touch like I should. The same goes for my close circle of friends. To my parents, Kathleen and Andre, thank you for showing me what real love looks like and for supporting all my hopes, dreams, and aspirations. And to Richard, thank you for your unwavering support, love, friendship, and for putting up with my crazy behind on a daily basis. You'll always be a great man in my eyes :) Also, thank you to Dr. Scantlebury for being a constant inspiration, in addition to your continued your mentorship and friendship.

To everyone who has ever believed in me or helped me in some form, I appreciate you more than you will ever know. And to everyone reading this book, thank you for taking the time out of your busy lives to read what I have to say. I hope this book has inspired each one of you to go out and reach for your dreams. Just don't forget to reach down and pull up those behind you as you reach for the stars and make it to the top.

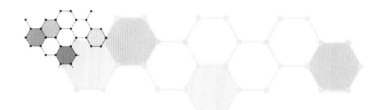

ABOUT THE AUTHOR

Dr. Danielle Ward received a BS degree in biochemistry (minor in chemistry) from Louisiana State University in 2009, a Master of Science degree in biochemistry from University of Saint Joseph in 2013, and her Doctor of Osteopathic Medicine degree from the Philadelphia College of Osteopathic Medicine - Georgia Campus in 2018. She then went on to complete a General Surgery Traditional Rotating Internship at Philadelphia College of Osteopathic Medicine in 2019.

Prior to working towards her medical degree, Dr. Ward took on a position as a full-time research associate at the LSU School of Veterinary Medicine where she worked for four years. She was involved in research focused on parasitology and immunology related to Neglected Tropical Diseases, and it led to her being included in articles published in well-regarded journals such as *Parasites & Vectors* and the *International Journal for Parasitology*.

While a full-time medical student, Dr. Ward balanced her time as a single mother to her elementary-aged daughter. Most notably, in 2016 she was the first osteopathic medical student to be elected as national president of the Student

National Medical Association (SNMA), and she went on to serve as the 2017-2018 SNMA National President. She also volunteered and managed to stay involved as a GA-PCOM Student Ambassador and with membership in various organizations. In 2013, Dr. Ward created the "Aspiring Minority Doctor" blog, which she actively maintains as documentation of her journey through medical school and beyond in addition to offering tips/advice to current pre-medical and medical students on similar paths. She has been featured on "Accepted.com", "Medical School Headquarters", the *Journal of the Student National Medical Association* (JSNMA), and in the *Atlanta Journal-Constitution*.

**If you would like to follow along on
Dr. Ward's journey, please check out her blog:**

www.aspiringminoritydoctor.com

Twitter: @minoritydoctor

Instagram: @minoritydoctor

Facebook: facebook.com/minoritydoctor

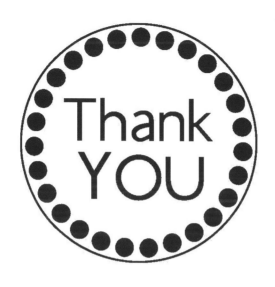

IF YOU ENJOYED
READING THIS BOOK,
PLEASE HELP ME OUT
BY LEAVING A
GLOWING AMAZON
REVIEW

Made in United States
Orlando, FL
29 May 2023

33605120R00090